DATE			

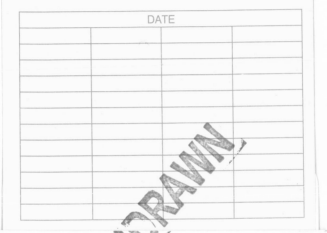

BAKER & TAYLOR

SHAME AND GUILT

EMOTIONS AND SOCIAL BEHAVIOR

Series Editor: Peter Salovey, Yale University

SHAME AND GUILT

JUNE PRICE TANGNEY
RONDA L. DEARING

Series Editor's Note by Peter Salovey

THE GUILFORD PRESS
New York   London

© 2002 The Guilford Press
A Division of Guilford Publications, Inc.
72 Spring Street, New York, NY 10012
www.guilford.com

Printed in the United States of America

This book is printed on acid-free paper.

Last digit is print number: 9   8   7   6   5   4   3   2   1

Library of Congress Cataloging-in-Publication Data

Tangney, June Price.
  Shame and guilt / June Price Tangney and Ronda L. Dearing.
    p. cm. — (Emotions and social behavior)
  Includes bibliographical references and index.
  ISBN 1-57230-715-3
    1. Shame. 2. Guilt. I. Dearing, Ronda L. II. Title. III. Series.

BF575.S45 T36 2002
  152.4—dc21   2001050143

To my intellectual "Dads,"
Joseph Masling and Seymour Feshbach
—J. P. T.

To my family,
for their ongoing encouragement and support
—R. L. D.

ABOUT THE AUTHORS

June Price Tangney, PhD, is Professor of Psychology at George Mason University. As an undergraduate, she worked with Dr. Joseph Masling at SUNY, Buffalo, and completed her doctorate in clinical psychology from the University of California–Los Angeles under the direction of Dr. Seymour Feshbach. Coeditor, with Kurt W. Fischer, of *Self-Conscious Emotions: The Psychology of Shame, Guilt, Embarrassment, and Pride,* she is currently Associate Editor for *Self and Identity,* and Consulting Editor for *Journal of Personality and Social Psychology, Personality and Social Psychology Bulletin, Psychological Assessment,* and *Journal of Personality.* Her research has been funded by the National Institute of Child Health and Human Development and the John Templeton Foundation.

Ronda L. Dearing, PhD, is a Postdoctoral Associate at the Research Institute on Addictions in Buffalo, New York. She became involved in the study of shame and guilt during her graduate training in clinical psychology at George Mason University, while working as a research assistant with June Tangney. Prior to her training in psychology, she worked as a medical technologist. Her doctoral dissertation focused on predictors of psychotherapy help seeking in therapists-in-training. More recent interests include help seeking in substance abuse, substance abuse treatment approaches, and the influence of shame-proneness on substance use.

SERIES EDITOR'S NOTE

One of the most enjoyable aspects of being the Series Editor for Guilford's Emotions and Social Behavior series is that I occasionally have the opportunity to shepherd to publication a book by an old friend. Such is the case for this latest volume in the series, *Shame and Guilt*, by my dear friend June Price Tangney (cowritten with Ronda L. Dearing). June and I have known each other for nearly 15 years, although we suspect that we encountered each other closer to 30 years ago as students in the same cohort at rival high schools in the suburbs of Buffalo, New York. As fellow clinical psychologists by training, but social psychologists by professional identification, I have always felt that Dr. Tangney and I shared a similar fondness for the rigorous empirical exploration of social processes in ecologically interesting contexts. No doubt, you will also share my enthusiasm for her cutting-edge approach to the emotions of shame and guilt, their relationship to each other, and their vastly different consequences for one's sense of self.

The book's analysis of shame and guilt, respectively, begins with a difference in emphasis. Shame is focused on a failing in the self ("Look what *I've* done"), but guilt focuses on morally disappointing behavior ("Look what I've *done*"). This distinction is rooted in the theorizing of the late Helen Block Lewis, an inspiring teacher during my graduate education at Yale. Given this distinction, it should not be surprising that while guilt can motivate individuals to try to behave in especially prosocial ways in order to expiate it, shame can induce intense rage as one experiences a threatened and diminished sense of self. From this starting point, June Tangney and Ronda Dearing provide a host of insights about the conceptualization and measurement of shame and guilt, their phenomenology, and the social consequences of these profoundly disturbing emotions. You will find this volume quite stimulating, especially if you are already familiar with this series and have read Mark R. Leary and Robin M. Kowalski's inspiring analysis in *Social Anxiety* and/or Rowland S. Miller's charming musings in *Embarrassment: Poise and Peril in Everyday Life*. I know that you will discover this book to be just as intriguing.

PETER SALOVEY, PhD
Chris Argyris Professor and Chair of Psychology
Yale University

ACKNOWLEDGMENTS

We owe a great intellectual debt to Yale psychologist Helen Block Lewis, the quintessential scientist–practitioner who—long before it was in vogue—combined keen clinical observations with the rigors of psychological theory and empirical research. The result, in 1971, was an entirely new conceptualization of shame and guilt—one which formed the foundation for our research. Helen died in 1987, but her work lives on.

June Price Tangney

I would like to thank the many teachers, colleagues, and students who have shaped my thinking over the years. I'm grateful to those who enriched my years as an undergraduate at SUNY, Buffalo, especially Jim Sawusch, who taught my undergraduate course in research methods; Irving Biederman, who gave me my first job and introduced me to my husband; and Joseph Masling, who was amazingly generous with his time, warmth and wisdom, mentoring a fledgling undergraduate. My graduate years at UCLA were nothing less than exhilarating. I'm especially grateful to Seymour and Norma Feshbach for their warmth, humor, support, and countless intellectual gifts. As my primary advisor, Sy instilled in me the importance of using flexible scientific methods to address pressing social issues. Norma has served as a model, teaching me how to tackle intriguing, but elusive, emotional processes and wrestle them to the ground. My first two years of teaching, at Bryn Mawr College, were pivotal. Bryn Mawr was the birthplace of our measures of shame and guilt, many thanks to my students and collaborators Susanne Burggraf, Barbara Domingos, and Hanne Hamme. And this work was further enhanced by much-needed guidance and encouragement from the chair, Rob Wozniak, and my colleague Mary Rohrkemper McCaislin. The vast majority of the work summarized in this volume was conducted over the past 13 years at George Mason University, in a remarkably collegial and intellectually rich department. I wish to thank Patricia Wagner especially, who as a first-year graduate student helped establish our lab; Ronda Dearing, who made this long journey of writing a delightful intellectual adventure; my dear friends and colleagues Jim Maddux and Susanne Denham; and two truly inspired chairs, Bob Smith and Jane Flinn.

Finally, I'm most thankful for the love and support of my family. I'm eternally grateful for my wonderful mother, Roberta Schauer, and my father, James Price. Among the countless gifts from my husband, John, I've benefited greatly from his deep appreciation for the value of data, his sound advice, and his delightful sense of humor. And I've cherished every interruption from my children—Erica, Lauren, and Ian.

Ronda L. Dearing

Most importantly, I would like to thank June Tangney, for being a wonderful mentor, friend, and source of intellectual growth and emotional support, as well as for providing me the unparalleled opportunity to work with her on this project. In addition, I would like to thank my family for their love and encouragement over the years and for helping me to believe that I could accomplish my goals. More specifically, sincere thanks to Ron and Barbara Dearing, and Craig and Maureen Dearing for providing numerous rejuvenating vacations at the lake. Many thanks to Gena and Dale Wolfson for providing wonderful hospitality when I need to escape to California. Thank you to Rachel, Sara, and Jack for your youthful vitality that allows me to be a kid sometimes. Other sources of friendship, support, and encouragement include Jenn and Paul Moosman, Frank McGinn and Susan Becelia, Deb Hill-Barlow, Kerry Gantt and Barbara Collier, Bryan Moosman, Carol Sacks, Ed Suarez, and Richard Cowles. I am also grateful to Candi Reinsmith, Angie Luzio, Deb Sinek, and Julie Borenstein. They have been a constant source of friendship, support, hard work, and fun. And finally, to all of my other teachers, supervisors, and friends, who helped me survive . . . thank you.

We both wish to thank the many graduate and undergraduate students who have worked in our lab over the years: Tania Abi-Najm, Gayathri Adikesavan, Kauser Ahmed, Cecilia Anon, Jalmeen Arora, Chris Arra, Brian Athey, Dee Dee Atkinson-Furr, Judy Back, Deb Hill-Barlow, Sheri Bailey, Ruth Barrientos, Rebecca Beam, Mary Bolton, Angie Boone, Eleni Boosalis, Elly Bordeaux, Julie Borenstein, Laura Bowling, Thea Bowling, Adam Brode, Phyllis Brodie, Crystal Brothers, Rachel Burroughs, Hannah Bustamante, Daniela Butler, Phyllis Byrne, Rhonda Campagna, Solange Caovan, Meredith Cato, Tina Chan, David Choi, Margaret Claustro, Luis Clavijo, Sarah Clements, Eddie Codel, Bill Connell, Lisa Conner, Joe Constantin, Kenny Corson, Susan Cottrell, Michelle Covert, Brit Creelman, Helena Crick, Sheila Cunningham, Ingrid Czintos, Chrissy Dale, Devra Dang, Zermarie Deacon, Steve Devers, Rosangela Di Manto, Robin Dold, Bertille Donohoe, Andy Drake, Leigh Earley, Keesha Edwards, Rebekka Eilers, Pam Estilong, Daniela Ettlinger, Barbara Evans, Kate Federline, Michelle Flanagan, Naheed Flanagan, Carey Fletcher, Laura Flicker, Bridget Fonseca, Kerry Ford, Faye Fortunato, Marcelle Fozard, Rebecca Frederick, Karen Friedman, Juan Funes, Emi Furukawa, John Gavlas, Jennifer Gosselin, Lynne Glikbarg, Richard Gramzow, Theresa Grant, Beth Gunzelman, Alice Hansburger, Barbara Harding, Bill Harman, Sharie Harman, Mark Hastings, Kim Havenner, Marna Hayes, Ashley Heald, Nancy Heleno, Charlie Hendricks, Jolene Hering, Junellyn Hood, Leslie Hughes, Kevin Hunt, Mark Hyer, Miguel Iglesias, Rebecca Jackson, Tricia Jacobsen, Christina James, Margaret Jefferies, Charlotte Joelsson, Heather Johnson, Karen Johnson, Mark Johnson, Caydie Jones, Heather Jones, Sahair Kaboli-Monfared, Ramineh Kangarloo, Marc Kaplan, Lesley Kato, Stephanie Kendall, Amy Kiernan, Nicole Kierein, Leslie Kirk, Linda Knauss, Greg Kramer, Stephanie Kowal, Chris Krause, Maria Lacayo, Allan Langley, Patrick Lechleitner, Norman Lee, Elizabeth Leon, Pete Lielbriedis, Conrad Loprete, Charmaine Lowe, Harry Malik, Terri Markel, Donna Marschall, Luis Mateus, James Maxfield, Amy McLaughlin, Patrick Meyer, Natalie Migliorini, Tim Mohr, Joanne Moller, Julie Morig, Corkie Morrill, Amy Muntz, Melody Myers, Yvette Nageotte, Thuy Nguyen, Jean No, Kyle Novak, Windi Oehms, Judy Okawa, Gabriel Ortiz, Troy Pafenberg, Gita Parlier, Caite Partamian, Elizabeth Patchen, Ray Payton, Chad Peddie, Phillip Pegg, Julie Pelch, Geoffrey

Pennoyer, Enrique Peralta, Marc Perez, Jill Perkins, Erica Perry, Amy Peterson, Dave Petersen, Greg Petrecca, Heather Phillips, Kayla Pope, Steve Potter, Michelle Price, Adam Rabinowitz, Sara Rahai, Paula Raikkonen, Michael Raumer, Candi Reinsmith, Justin Reznick, Diana Rodriguez, Fernando Rodriquez, Lori Roop, Karen Rosenberg, Tricia Roy, Karey Rush, Gary Russell, Provie Rydstrom, Paul Saenz, Leila Safavian, Dolly Saini, Jackie Sakati, Veronica Sanchez, Jennifer Sanftner, Ann Scharff, Heather Sevier, Vicki Shaffer, Ann Shannon, Gordon Shaw, Kay Shows, Farhad Siahpoush, Deb Sinek, Chris Smart, Erika Smith, Steve Smith, Caryn Smonskey, Jonathan Sollinger, Larry Spahr, Gary Stone, Stephanie Storck, Dave Testa, Rebecca Thompson, Chris Tiller, Andrea Thorson, Tammy Tower, Mike Tragakis, Berrin Tutuncuoplu, Tony Tzoumas, Kim Udell, Lisa Unrine, Jocelyn Valenzuela, Suchi Vatsa, Jennifer Vaught, Svenja Wacker, Patti Wagner, Kristine Welch, Tammy Walker, Abigail Wear, Dina Wieczynski, Rebecca Wilbur, Tara Williams, Simone Whyte, Sabura Woods, Susan Wyman, Tim Yerington, Siyon Yi, Nancy Zenich, and Tev Zukor. This has truly been a collaborative venture that benefited greatly from each student's contribution.

Much of the research summarized in this volume was supported by research grants from the National Institute of Child Health and Human Development, the John Templeton Foundation, the National Institutes of Health, the National Science Foundation, and George Mason University. Many thanks to the program managers and reviewers who helped make this research happen.

We also offer sincere thanks to our ever-patient and supportive publisher, Seymour Weingarten, and Series Editor, Peter Salovey. And we owe a great debt of gratitude to Gary Stone, Beth Gunzelman, and Doris Yuspeh for their administrative support and much-needed sense of humor through countless drafts and reference checks. Many thanks also to Bert Zelman of Publishers Workshop, Inc., and Anna Nelson of The Guilford Press for the terrific editorial work, and to Mark Leary for providing invaluable comments and suggestions on an earlier draft.

Finally, we extend our warmest thanks to the many children, parents, grandparents, teachers, undergraduates, airport travelers, and others who have so generously participated in our research over the years. With your help, we have learned much about the dynamics of shame and guilt.

CONTENTS

Chapter 1

WHAT IS SO IMPORTANT ABOUT SHAME AND GUILT?

"Your soul is like a sacred, holy book," our nun explained on a gray Monday afternoon, preparing us for our first-grade First Confession. "Because of Christ's terrible sacrifice, you are born with a beautiful pure white soul, shining with goodness. Each page is clean, holy, and pristine." As a 6-year-old, I didn't know what "pristine" meant, but I knew it was good. I warmed to the idea of having the gift of such a beautiful white soul. The image was crisp and vivid. "But!" the nun thundered, shattering the mood, "each time you sin—even the littlest sin—you get a GREAT Big Black BLOT on one of those pages. And you may go to confession, God may forgive you, but that ugly black blot never goes away."

My heart fell. I began imagining all the blots already there on my little soul—marring its God-given beauty forever. As a 6-year-old, with two younger brothers, I'd already had my fair share of fights, of envy, of anger. I could remember bending the truth with my parents, selfishly grabbing the last cupcake, misbehaving at my grandparents' house. The list went on. I had a soul already marked, soiled, unworthy.

Another message I gleaned from Sunday sermons, stories of saints, and Monday afternoon religious education classes was that: To be a good person, you have to feel *really* bad. If you're not a saint, if you occasionally, inevitably sin, then your worthiness and closeness to God hinges on how bad you feel about those sins. Good people feel intense remorse and regret, and a painful, grinding self-scrutiny and denouncement of the self. Bad people just brush it off. They might feel a twinge of remorse. But good people don the hair shirt—and suffer.

From what I gather, these messages are not part of the official Catholic doctrine.[1] But they are the messages I received, as interpreted by important socialization figures—our parish priests and nuns, my parents, aunts and uncles—and which I then filtered and pieced

1

together with the unsophisticated mind of a child. *The better a person you are, the worse you'll feel.* Talk about a dilemma! What an unattractive goal to strive toward!

One of the most hopeful and gratifying conclusions to come out of our 12 years of research on shame and guilt is that that notion of morality is wrong. Dead wrong. You don't have to feel *really* bad to be a good person. In fact, if anything, the data suggest to the contrary. In the realm of moral emotions, more is not necessarily better. Moderately painful feelings of guilt about specific behaviors motivate people to behave in a moral, caring, socially responsible manner. In contrast, intensely painful feelings of shame do *not* appear to steer people in a constructive, moral direction. Such intense moral pain about the self cuts to our core, exacting a heavy "penance" perhaps. But rather than motivating reparative action, shame often motivates denial, defensive anger and aggression.

—JUNE PRICE TANGNEY

Shame and guilt are rich human emotions that serve important functions at both the individual and relationship levels. On the one hand, as moral emotions, shame and guilt are among our most private, intimate experiences. In the face of transgression or error, the self turns toward the self—evaluating and rendering judgment. Thus, the experience of shame or guilt can guide our behavior and influence who we are in our own eyes. On the other hand, shame and guilt are inextricably linked to the self in relationship with others. These emotions develop from our earliest interpersonal experiences—in the family and in other key relationships. And throughout the lifespan, these emotions exert a profound and continued influence on our behavior in interpersonal contexts. Shame and guilt are thus both "self-conscious" and "moral" emotions: self-conscious in that they involve the self evaluating the self, and moral in that they presumably play a key role in fostering moral behavior.

Shame and guilt have captured the attention of clinical, social, and developmental psychologists for generations. As a consequence, there is a rich and varied theoretical literature pertaining to these moral emotions—a literature that includes psychodynamic, cognitive, and developmental perspectives. But it is only recently that psychologists have begun systematic empirical research on the nature and implications of shame and guilt. The gap between the theoretical and empirical treatment of these emotions has been due largely to difficulties in the measurement of shame and guilt. These are difficult constructs to assess, first, because they are exclusively internal phenomena that are not amenable to direct observation and, second, because people do not typically have a clear sense of the distinction between shame and guilt, which poses problems for introspective accounts. In recent years, however, a number of researchers have tackled the measurement challenge, and there is now emerging a "critical mass" of scientifically based knowledge pertaining to the emotions of shame and guilt. So in contrast to the psychoanalytically oriented books on shame that have appeared in recent years (e.g., Goldberg, 1991; Jacoby, 1991; Lansky & Morrison, 1997; H. B. Lewis, 1987d; Miller, 1996; A. P. Morrison, 1989, 1996; Nathanson, 1987b), this book highlights recent empirical findings from our own lab and from colleagues in the fields of clinical, social, personality, and developmental psychology.

We have chosen to emphasize the role of shame and guilt in interpersonal relationships throughout this book because we think this is one of the most exciting and robust themes emerging from the current research. The research of the first author took a fairly dramatic turn in this direction early on. Tangney recalls, "When I first began studying shame and guilt, I had thought that my work would be primarily concerned with the implications of these emotions for psychopathology— particularly depression. And while this has been a fruitful area of inquiry, one of the most consistent themes emerging from virtually every study in our lab is that shame and guilt have important and quite different implications for interpersonal relationships."

In brief, shame is an extremely painful and ugly feeling that has a negative impact on interpersonal behavior. Shame-prone individuals appear relatively more likely to blame others (as well as themselves) for negative events, more prone to a seething, bitter, resentful kind of anger and hostility, and less able to empathize with others in general. Guilt, on the other hand, may not be that bad after all. Guilt-prone individuals appear better able to empathize with others and to accept responsibility for negative interpersonal events. They are relatively less prone to anger than their shame-prone peers—but when angry, these individuals appear more likely to express their anger in a fairly direct (and one might speculate, more constructive) manner. This is an intriguing pattern, and it is the aspect of shame and guilt that has the most direct applied implications—for parents, teachers, and clinicians alike.

The book's intended audience is fairly broad, including professionals in social psychology, clinical psychology and psychiatry, developmental psychology, and sociology, as well as interested nonspecialists and laypersons. The volume is unique in its focus on empirical approaches to the study of shame and guilt and in its reliance on a range of theoretical perspectives. Thus, it is a valuable source for the growing number of researchers interested in the study of affect and social behavior. At the same time, many of the issues have quite clear applied implications. Although the book is empirically based, we have made a concerted effort to present the material in a readable style that underlines the practical implications of findings related to the moral emotions. For example, unnecessary technical detail has been excluded from the body of the text, and interested readers are referred to appendices and other published reports.

ORGANIZATION AND CONTENT

We begin in Chapter 2 with an in-depth discussion of the phenomenology of shame and guilt. One of the most frequent questions we encounter is whether shame and guilt really are different emotions. This chapter presents a summary of research findings clearly indicating that shame and guilt are distinct affective experiences, each with their own contrasting motivational and behavioral manifestations.

Chapter 3 focuses on the assessment of shame and guilt. Much of our work and the work of others has been concerned with the styles or dispositions—proneness to shame and proneness to guilt. These are difficult constructs to assess, and it is largely the problem of measurement that has impeded empirical study of shame and guilt until recently. In this chapter, we review the range of approaches that have been developed for measuring proneness to shame and guilt, commenting on their relative strengths and weaknesses. In addition, because our measures were used in many of the studies to be highlighted in subsequent chapters, we will describe in some detail the development of the Tests of Self-Conscious Affect (TOSCA for adults, TOSCA-A for adolescents, and TOSCA-C for children), and their precursors, the Self-Conscious Affect and Attribution Inventories. Copies of these measures, with relevant psychometric data, appear in Appendix B. We also grapple with the challenges involved in assessing feelings of shame and guilt "in the moment."

Chapter 4 explores the implications of shame and guilt for the self. We have chosen to focus on this aspect of shame and guilt early in the book because we believe that the dynamics of shame and guilt in interpersonal relationships can be understood only with reference to how shame and guilt affect self-esteem and related self functions. In particular, it seems likely that the painful global self-focus of shame renders the self vulnerable to a range of difficulties, which then have a negative impact on interpersonal behavior and functioning.

Chapter 5 examines shame and guilt as they relate to interpersonal empathy. We summarize research showing that the shame-prone person is not an empathic person. Shame-proneness is generally negatively correlated with empathy, whereas guilt-proneness is generally positively associated with empathy. It appears that the focus of guilt on specific behaviors facilitates an other-oriented empathic connection whereas the painful self-focus of shame seems to impede sensitivity to others.

In Chapter 6, we turn to what we see as one of the most exciting results from our studies thus far—the differential relation of shame and guilt to hostility and anger. The results across studies are quite consistent: guilt-proneness is negligibly or negatively correlated with indices of anger, hostility, and aggression. In contrast, we have observed a strong and consistent link between shame and measures of anger and hostility. This finding that anger is differentially related to shame and guilt was a real empirical "discovery" for us; that is, it came directly from our data. Shamed people are not only prone to anger, they are also inclined to express their anger in nonconstructive ways. In contrast, guilt motivates individuals to accept responsibility, and may actually inhibit interpersonal anger and hostility. In Chapter 10, we follow up on the implications of these results, speculating that the shame–anger dynamic may be particularly important in close interpersonal relationships and that this dynamic may be a key feature in instances of domestic violence.

Chapter 7 examines the differential relation of shame and guilt to psychological symptoms, particularly depression. We suggest that people can respond to the devastating pain of shame in two very different ways: the shamed individual can become angry at the world, attempting to shift the blame onto others, as indicated in Chapter 6; or the shamed individual can withdraw from others, holding in or internalizing the shame, and thereby becoming vulnerable to a host of psychological symptoms, especially depression. Research consistently shows a link between proneness to shame and a range of symptom clusters. Further, although shame-proneness is clearly related to a depressogenic attributional style, shame-proneness accounts for a substantial portion of variance in depression, above and beyond that accounted for by attributional style. There is much more controversy regarding the relationship of guilt to psychopathology. Studies employing adjective checklist-type (and other globally worded) measures of shame and guilt have found that both shame-prone and guilt-prone styles are associated with psychological symptoms. On the other hand, a very different pattern of results emerges when scenario-based measures are used that are sensitive to the distinction between shame about the self versus guilt about a specific behavior. Across studies of both children and adults, the tendency to experience "shame-free" guilt is essentially unrelated to psychological symptoms. In Chapter 11, we discuss how an explicit consideration of shame-related issues may be useful in the treatment of a number of psychological and interpersonal problems.

Chapter 8 examines the link between shame and guilt and moral behavior. Shame and guilt are considered by many to be, first and foremost, "moral emotions" because they presumably represent powerful internal sanctions against socially and morally unacceptable behavior. It is ironic, then, that so little research has addressed this issue directly. In Chapter 8, we summarize results from an ongoing longitudinal study showing that shame-proneness assessed in the fifth grade predicts later high school suspension, hard drug use, and suicide attempts. In contrast, guilt-prone fifth graders were more likely to later apply to college and do community service. They were less likely to make suicide attempts, to use heroin, or to drive under the influence of alcohol and drugs, and they began drinking at a later age. Guilt-prone fifth graders were less likely to be arrested, convicted, and incarcerated. In adolescence they had fewer sexual partners and were more likely to practice "safe sex" and use birth control.

Chapter 9 takes a closer look at the development of shame and guilt. First, we examine normative developmental changes in the experience of shame and guilt. Shame emerges first, at about age 2, whereas guilt requires more sophisticated cognitive abilities not typically seen much before age 8. Studies of children, adolescents, and adults also suggest ongoing developmental changes in the nature of the shame and guilt experience. In Chapter 9 we also consider at length the development of individual differences in moral emotional style. What individual, family, and other social factors help shape children's emerging tendencies to experience shame and guilt? What can parents do to foster an "optimal" moral emotional style; for example, can we pinpoint specific disciplinary strategies that encourage an adaptive capacity for guilt versus maladaptive shame reactions? (In Chapter 12, we discuss the applied implications of these findings for parents and teachers who work on a day-to-day basis to raise morally competent children.)

Chapter 10 explores shame and guilt in intimate relationships. We look at gender differences in communication styles, couples' conflict, and the important role of shame in sexual relationships. Feelings of shame appear to be especially relevant in the context of safe sex practices (and the potential spread of sexually transmitted diseases), spouse abuse, and being a sexual minority. Throughout the chapter, we discuss everyday situations in which knowledge of the shame dynamic can enhance our sensitivity and effectiveness in relationships with spouses, friends, and colleagues.

Chapters 11 and 12 focus on the applied implications of shame and guilt. In Chapter 11 we discuss the implications of moral emotions in psychotherapy. For the clinician, shame and guilt play a role both in the understanding and treatment of psychological symptoms (e.g., depression, domestic violence), and in management of the therapeutic process itself. For example, as H. B. Lewis (1971) has noted, shame-related reactions very likely account for many failures in treatment, including pervasive resistance and premature termination of therapy. In developing a "third ear" for shame-related processes, the therapist can enhance his or her effectiveness with many clients, particularly those who are prone to shame. Regarding symptomotology (as discussed in Chapters 6 and 7), research indicates that some of the most common presenting problems are likely to be, at least in part, shame-based. Chapter 12 discusses the implications of shame and guilt for parents, teachers, and society. Shame and guilt are part and parcel of both parenting and teaching. In this chapter, we discuss the dynamics of shame and guilt at home and in the classroom, and we provide empirically based recommendations for enhancing children's moral and emotional development. We also consider the implications of shame and guilt for our criminal justice system. We believe that in each of these domains, recognition of the distinction between shame and guilt is an important first step in making ours a more moral society.

OVERARCHING THEMES

Woven throughout the book are several "meta-themes" worth emphasizing at the outset. First, we want to repeatedly underscore how critical it is to distinguish between shame about the self versus guilt about specific behaviors. Across multiple domains, the correlates of shame are in a direction *opposite* that of guilt. Failure to note this divergence, particularly when an investigator is conducting research, can result in downright erroneous conclusions. For the researcher, the mechanics of statistics guarantee that substantial, but divergent correlates of shame and guilt—each of practical importance—will cancel each other out, yielding the appearance of *no* relationship to other constructs. For the clinician, parent, or spouse, the shame and guilt distinction is similarly important for understanding human behavior. As this book repeatedly illustrates, the dynamics, motivations, and behaviors associated with these oft-confused emotions move people in very different directions— guilt typically for the better, and shame typically for the worse.

Another matter we want to stress is the importance of collecting data. Throughout the book, we point out "surprises" that have turned up through careful empirical inquiry into shame and guilt dynamics in real life. As in so many other areas of psychology, the findings are not merely an empirical demonstration of what "everybody already knows." For example, a number of judges across the United States routinely employ "shaming sentences," based on the mistaken assumption that shame fosters repentance and reform. Systematic empirical research importantly informs our understanding of human nature, often in very practical ways.

Reflecting our belief in the importance of research evidence, we have chosen to include actual data at strategic points throughout the book to give the reader a flavor of the nature and scope of data supporting our conclusions. For example, we have included tables summarizing a variety of studies on shame and guilt to give readers an opportunity to evaluate the level of support for our assertions and to draw their own conclusions accordingly. Readers who are less interested in this detailed information may skip the tables, correlations, and other technical material. We have made every effort to summarize the main points in the text, in language geared toward nonspecialists. Thus, we hope that the book is comprehensive and yet accessible to a broad audience.

A final issue is more conceptual than practical. One message from this book is that guilt and especially shame lurk in corners we never imagined. These are powerful, ubiquitous emotions that come into play across most important areas of life. But shame is not at the root of everything. One of our long-standing concerns is the problem of treating shame as an "elastic construct," as is especially likely among theorists who endorse H. B. Lewis's (1971) notion of "by-passed" shame. In some accounts, shame masquerades so frequently as anger, depression, anxiety, and discomfort that it seems all the world's a shame! In the extreme, this perspective suggests that shame is everywhere, everything is caused by shame, and shame is at the root of every negative interaction. Not all episodes of anger are based in shame. People become anxious, they avoid uncomfortable situations, they giggle, for many different reasons. While we agree that the importance of shame is often overlooked in many contexts, there is a danger in overgeneralizing as well. At some point, the construct (and measurement) of shame needs to be distinct from other constructs if we are to meaningfully study the relationship of shame to anything else.

We hope that readers will enjoy this journey charting the moral emotions and will come away with an understanding of shame and guilt that is both personally and professionally valuable.

NOTE

1. And, as it turns out, religious background is relatively unimportant in determining a person's propensity to experience shame and guilt. See Chapter 9 for a more detailed discussion of the impact of religion on moral emotions.

Chapter 2

WHAT IS THE DIFFERENCE BETWEEN SHAME AND GUILT?

"Shame is regret.
 Guilt is sin-regret."

"Shame is when you know you did something wrong and you're sorry
    you did it.
 Guilt is when you did something that was wrong and you can't admit
    it."

"Shame is a feeling that you have when your not happy of your
    individual outcome or a certain matter.
 Guilt is when you've done something you felt you shouldn't have."

"Shame is the feeling that everyone else thinks you have done wrong
    and all know what you have done.
 Guilt is the feeling that you know what you have done and by your
    standards it is wrong."

"Shame is when one has done something which contradicts their own
    morals or beliefs.
 Guilt is when one has gone against their true nature."

"Shame is feeling guilty.
 Guilt is feeling ashamed about something."

These are some of the answers we received from a group of college undergraduates when we asked them to define the words "shame" and "guilt" and describe the difference between the two emotions. Obviously, they did not do very well. For the most part, these bright, well-educated young adults could not provide consistent, meaningful definitions of these common human emotions. The big surprise was that when we asked college students to describe and rate *specific, personal* shame and guilt experiences, their ratings of these emotion experiences differed in consistent, theoretically meaningful ways. In other words, it appeared that these college students "knew more than they could say" about shame and guilt. As we describe in greater detail later in this chapter, their ratings of personal shame and guilt events strongly indicate that they, in fact, experience these as quite distinct emotions. But when asked to define these emotions in the abstract, the students really couldn't articulate any consistent clear differences between shame and guilt.

College students aren't unique in this regard. A quick review of the psychological literature shows that the "experts," too, often use the terms shame and guilt inconsistently or interchangeably. For example, psychologists frequently mention shame and guilt in the same breath, as moral emotions that help people choose the high moral road (e.g., Damon, 1988; Eisenberg, 1986; Harris, 1989; Schulman & Mekler, 1985), or as potentially problematic emotions that can cause any one of a number of psychological problems (Fossum & Mason, 1986; Potter-Efron, 1989; Rodin, Silberstein, & Striegel-Moore, 1985). In the clinical literature, especially, it is not uncommon to see psychologists refer to "feelings of shame and guilt" or to discuss the "effects of shame and guilt" without making any distinction between the two emotions.

In everyday conversations, people typically avoid the term "shame." In fact, one could easily argue that today's U.S. society is rather "shame-phobic." The average person rarely speaks of his or her own "shame." Instead, people refer to "guilt" (e.g., "I felt so *guilty* when I realized what an inconsiderate person I've been") when they mean they felt shame, guilt, or some combination of the two.

Recent theory and research, however, has identified important differences between these two closely related emotions—differences that appear to have rather profound implications both for psychological adjustment and for social behavior. In this chapter, we describe several theoretical distinctions between shame and guilt that have been suggested by social scientists over the years. We begin with a review of early attempts to differentiate shame and guilt, including those based on psychoanalytic and anthropological theories. For example, a common basis for distinguishing between shame and guilt focuses on presumed differences in the types of *situations* that elicit these emotions. We then summarize recent empirical results that seriously challenge this assumption and we describe the empirical support for H. B. Lewis's (1971) reconceptualization, which emphasizes shame's focus on the self versus guilt's focus on specific behaviors.

EARLY DISTINCTIONS BETWEEN SHAME AND GUILT

Attempts to distinguish between shame and guilt are not new. Some of the most influential distinctions between the two emotions date back many decades, from psychoanalytic circles and from anthropology. Although recent empirical research has not provided much support for these earlier views, it is useful to be aware of these perspectives because they can be found, in one form or another, in both the psychological and popular literatures. In fact, in our research we saw evidence of these earlier notions of how shame and guilt differ in the definitions provided by some of our more articulate college students.

The Psychoanalytic Perspective

Over the years, psychoanalytically oriented theories have probably paid the most attention to shame and guilt. But the father of psychoanalysis, Sigmund Freud, too, largely neglected the distinction between these two emotions. In his earlier work, Freud (1905/1953b) briefly discussed shame as a reaction formation against sexually exhibitionistic impulses. From this early perspective, feelings of shame were invoked to defend against desires to publicly call attention to oneself sexually. But in his later writings (Freud, 1914/1957, 1923/1961d, 1924/1961c, 1925/1961b) he essentially ignored the construct of shame, focusing instead on a rather cognitive concept of guilt in relation to superego conflicts. According to Freud, feelings of guilt arise when id or ego impulses or behaviors clash with the moral standards of the superego (see H. B. Lewis, 1971, N. K. Morrison, 1987, and Tangney, 1994, for more detailed analyses of Freud's approach to shame and guilt). Lewis (1971) has argued that in developing a theory that focused almost exclusively on guilt, Freud (like many contemporary psychologists) may have mislabeled his patients' shame experiences as guilt experiences.

A number of post-Freudian theorists made explicit attempts to distinguish between shame and guilt within a neo-Freudian framework (e.g., Hartmann & Loewenstein, 1962; Jacobson, 1954; Piers & Singer, 1953). Fairly early in his writings, Freud (1914/1957) introduced the notion of an "ego-ideal." Although Freud largely abandoned this construct in his later work, subsequent ego psychologists picked up on this theme and elaborated on the distinction between ego-ideal (roughly, an idealized moral self) and superego (or conscience) proper. A number of theorists applied this distinction to their conceptualization of shame and guilt. For example, Piers and Singer (1953) viewed guilt as a reaction to clashes between the ego and the superego (with its roots in fears of castration, similar to Freud's own notions). In contrast, shame was conceptualized as a reaction to clashes between the ego and the ego-ideal (with its roots in feelings of inferiority, and consequent fears of loss of love and abandonment). This neo-Freudian distinction between shame and guilt can be seen as a precursor of H. B. Lewis's (1971) later distinction between self concerns and behavior concerns, and it is consistent with Erikson's (1950) descriptions of shame as global exposed self-doubt versus guilt over misguided behavior (initiative). But the neo-Freudian structural distinction is not without its problems. For example, Hartmann and Loewenstein (1962) questioned the practical utility of such a structural distinction. And, more recently, Lindsay-Hartz (1984) provided evidence apparently contradicting Piers and Singer (1953), showing that shame typically results from a *negative* ideal (e.g., the recognition that "We are who we do not want to be"), rather than from a recognition that we have failed to live up to some *positive* ego-ideal.

With the emergence of self psychology, shame gained an even more prominent place in psychodynamic theory. Quite a number of psychoanalytically oriented theorists have cited shame as a major factor in a range of psychological disorders (Kohut, 1971; A. P. Morrison, 1989; N. K. Morrison, 1987; Nathanson, 1987a, 1987b, 1987c). But in their new focus on shame, these theories tend to give short shrift to guilt. Ironically, in many cases, the construct of guilt (distinct from shame) is largely neglected and, as in traditional Freudian theory, the distinction between these two emotions has been lost.

The Anthropological Perspective

Outside of psychoanalytic circles, when people make a distinction between shame and guilt, they often refer to differences in the content and/or structure of events eliciting these emotions. The assumption here, popularized by mid-20th-century anthropologists (e.g., Benedict, 1946), is that certain *kinds of situations* lead to shame whereas other *kinds of situations* lead to guilt. For example, there is a long-standing notion that shame is a more "public" emotion than guilt. Shame is seen as arising from public exposure and disapproval of some shortcoming or transgression, whereas guilt is seen as a more "private" experience arising from self-generated pangs of conscience.

This public–private distinction remains a frequently cited basis for distinguishing between shame and guilt. Gehm and Scherer (1988), for example, speculated that "shame is usually dependent on the public exposure of one's frailty or failing, whereas guilt may be something that remains a secret with us, no one else knowing of our breach of social norms or of our responsibility for an immoral act" (p. 74).

As it turns out, there isn't much empirical support for this public–private distinction. In fact, results from several recent studies call into question this long-standing notion (Tangney, Marschall, Rosenberg, Barlow, & Wagner, 1994; Tangney, Miller, Flicker, & Barlow, 1996). For example, we conducted what appears to be the first systematic analysis of "audiences" to shame- and guilt-eliciting events (Tangney et al., 1994). In this study, we asked several hundred children and adults to describe recent events in which they had experienced shame, guilt, and pride. We then analyzed these narrative accounts of real-life emotion episodes to evaluate, among other things, just how public or private these events really were.

Our results clearly challenge the anthropologists' public–private distinction. Although shame and guilt were *both* most often experienced in the presence of others (among both children and adults), a substantial number of respondents reported shame experiences occurring alone—when *not* in the presence of others. More important, "solitary" shame was about as prevalent as "solitary" guilt (see Figure 2.1). Among children, 17.2% of shame narratives versus 14.9% of guilt narratives involved situations in which no other person was present. Among adults, 16.5% of shame episodes versus 22.5% of guilt episodes were experienced alone. (Pride was most likely to be experienced alone; 33.8% of the children and 25.5% of the adults reported solitary pride experiences.)

Even more to the point, we assessed whether or not anyone was explicitly aware of the respondent's behavior. This audience awareness variable represents the strongest test of Benedict's (1946) notion that

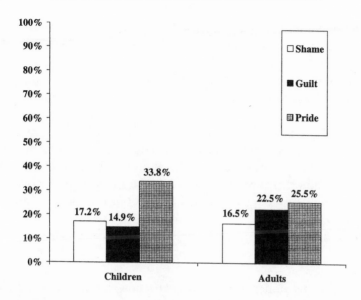

FIGURE 2.1. Percentage of "solitary" shame, guilt, and pride experiences.

shame is differentially related to public exposure or scrutiny, because it is possible that others may have been present in the situation but not aware of the respondent's behavior (e.g., a respondent telling a lie). Figure 2.2 shows the percentages of children's and adults' shame, guilt, and pride events in which others were clearly unaware of the respondent's behavior. For all three emotions, the large majority of situations involved audience awareness of the respondent's behavior. The only appreciable difference was between pride versus shame and guilt among adults. Adults perceived that others were more likely to be aware of their behavior in pride situations and somewhat less likely to be aware of their behavior in shame and guilt situations. Importantly, there was no difference in "audience awareness" when shame and guilt events were compared. In the accounts provided by both children and adults, others were no more likely to be aware of shame-inducing behaviors than they were of guilt-inducing behaviors, in contrast to the anthropologists' public–private distinction (e.g., Benedict, 1946).

Similarly, in a subsequent independent study of adults' narrative accounts of personal shame, guilt, and embarrassment experiences (Tangney, Miller, et al., 1996), there was no evidence that shame was the more "public" emotion. In fact, in this latter study, shame was somewhat *more* likely (18.2%) than guilt (10.4%) to occur outside of the presence of an observing audience.

For example, Rick,[1] a 21-year-old college student related this "solitary" shame experience:

> "When I was in junior high, my brother bought a *Penthouse* magazine and hid it in his closet. I found it, looked at it, then put it back. Somehow, my mother found it and yelled at my brother in front of me. She didn't know that I had looked at it. I was so ashamed that I looked at it (and frightened of getting yelled at) that I just sat there silently."

In contrast, 20-year-old Jesse described this very public guilt experience:

> "I was having dinner with a bunch of friends, and we were all jokingly teasing one of the friends. He's one of my best friends, and it was clear that this was all done in jest. Anyway, later on, after reflecting on the dinner, it occurred to me that he probably wasn't enjoying all the

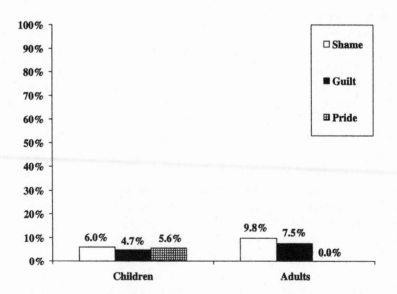

FIGURE 2.2. Percentage of shame, guilt, and pride experiences in which no one was aware of behavior.

teasing. I mentioned that to him, and he said he hadn't minded, but still I didn't feel very good about it—mild guilt."

Similarly, 26-year-old Anthony described a very public guilt episode:

"While growing up I ran with what would be considered a 'bad crowd' under peer pressure. I got caught by the police on weapons and narcotics charges. I had to go to court for the better part of a year. This made me feel extremely guilty since it was entirely against my parents' upbringing and expectations, as well as society's."

If shame and guilt do not differ in terms of the degree of public exposure, do they differ in terms of the *types* of the transgressions or failures that elicit them? Do certain kinds of behaviors give rise to shame, while other kinds of behaviors give rise to feelings of guilt? Not really, as it turns out. Our analyses of the personal shame and guilt experiences provided by both children and adults indicate that there are very few, if any, "classic" shame-inducing or guilt-inducing situations (Tangney, 1992; Tangney, Marschall, Rosenberg, Barlow, & Wagner, 1994). Most types of events (e.g., lying, cheating, stealing, failing to help another, disobeying parents) were cited by some people in connection with feelings of shame and by other people in connection with guilt. Unlike moral transgressions, which are equally likely to elicit shame or guilt, there was some evidence that nonmoral failures and shortcomings (e.g., socially inappropriate behavior or dress) may be more likely to elicit shame. Even so, failures in work, school, or sport settings and violations of social conventions were cited by a significant number of children and adults in connection with guilt (Tangney et al., 1994).

In short, there were strong parallels in the type of situation that caused shame and guilt in our research participants. For example, consider the similarities between 36-year-old Martin's guilt experience, "I ignored a street person asking for money," and Bianca's shame experience, "An elderly lady asked for a donation and I very quickly refused her, only to feel immediately ashamed for not having been more Christian and helpful." Another college student, Ahmed, related this guilt experience:

"I experienced guilt during college when I cheated on my girlfriend. She later found out, which escalated the tension that had previously existed."

Marilyn, a 38-year-old college student, related a similar situation when asked to describe a shame experience:

> "I felt ashamed of feeling I might like to have an extramarital affair. I never thought it would be me to consider this. I have not taken the plunge; however, the fact that I thought of it makes me feel shame."

HELEN BLOCK LEWIS'S (1971) RECONCEPTUALIZATION: SHAME AND GUILT DIFFER IN FOCUS ON SELF VERSUS BEHAVIOR

How do shame and guilt differ, then, if not in terms of the types of situations that elicit them? In 1971, Helen Block Lewis, a clinical psychologist at Yale University, presented a radically different and now highly influential distinction between these two emotions. In her landmark book *Shame and Guilt in Neurosis*, Lewis (1971) merged her extensive clinical background in psychoanalytic theory and ego psychology with ideas drawn from her experimental work with Herman A. Witkin on field-dependent versus field-independent cognitive styles. According to Lewis (1971), a key difference between shame and guilt centers on the role of the self in these experiences. She wrote: "The experience of shame is directly about the *self*, which is the focus of evaluation. In guilt, the self is not the central object of negative evaluation, but rather the *thing* done or undone is the focus. In guilt, the self is negatively evaluated in connection with something but is not itself the focus of the experience" (p. 30; emphasis in original).

Lewis (1971) proposed that this differential emphasis on self ("*I* did that horrible thing") versus behavior ("I *did* that horrible *thing*") leads to very different phenomenological experiences. She described shame as an acutely painful emotion that is typically accompanied by a sense of shrinking or of "being small" and by a sense of worthlessness and powerlessness. Shamed people also feel exposed. Although shame doesn't necessarily involve an actual observing audience that is present to witness one's shortcomings, there is often the imagery of how one's defective self would appear to others. Lewis (1971) described a split in self-functioning in which the self is both agent and object of observation and disapproval. An observing self witnesses and denigrates the focal self as unworthy and reprehensible. Finally, shame often leads to a desire to escape or to hide—to sink into the floor and disappear.

In contrast, Lewis (1971) viewed guilt as typically a less painful and devastating experience than shame because, in guilt, our primary concern is with a particular behavior, somewhat apart from the self. So guilt doesn't affect one's core identity or self-concept. Feelings of guilt can be painful nonetheless. Guilt involves a sense of tension, remorse, and regret over the "bad thing" done. People in the midst of a guilt experience often report a nagging focus or preoccupation with the transgression—thinking of it over and over, wishing they had behaved differently or could somehow undo the deed.

For example, 23-year-old Cecilia described this guilt experience:

> "I experienced guilt when one of the ministers asked me did I get my driver's license reinstated, and I told him 'Yes' because I had been driving and I didn't want him to know that I was disobeying the law. In about 4 days, we were in church preparing ourselves for communion, and the Holy Spirit had been convicting me so bad, I had to tell the minister the truth before even taking communion."

Cecilia's description of a personal guilt experience illustrates the nagging sense of tension and regret that is so characteristic of guilt. (The Holy Spirit—and Cecilia's conscience—apparently had been "convicting" this woman for four long days.) It also highlights the guilt's press toward confession, reparation, and apology. Cecilia's experience of guilt wasn't driving her to take further steps to hide her dishonesty. Rather, in her guilt, she felt compelled to take the more difficult path of telling her minister the truth.

Similarly, 18-year-old Tyrone described this recent guilt experience:

> "Last fall I got really sick at the beginning of the school semester. I missed the first month of classes and could not catch up. I had to withdraw from all but one class. When you withdraw, you don't get your money back. My mom and dad pay tuition, and they weren't real happy about losing $975. I felt guilty, so I got two jobs, worked 70 hours a week, and paid them back in 3 weeks."

In contrast, feelings of shame are more likely to motivate a desire to hide or escape the shame-inducing situation, as illustrated by 47-year-old Maria's description of an early shame experience:

> "When I was 6 years old, at the end of the kindergarten school year, I experienced shame. On the last day of school, only the older children

were expected to go to school, but my mother didn't know this and she sent me to school anyway. I knew the kindergartners were not expected that day. Since my mother insisted that I go, I thought, 'Well, maybe I am to get some kind of special prize for being such a good student. Maybe they are going to announce that I can skip the first grade.' When I got to school, one of the teachers saw me and said, 'Oh, you are not supposed to be here today!' *I turned around and ran all the way home, so ashamed that I had had these thoughts.*" [emphasis added]

Similarly, 20-year-old Janice described this shame experience:

"It was a piano recital that I really had no desire to take part in, since I get extremely nervous on such occasions. . . . I performed and messed up the whole thing in a serious way, in front of people I knew and who had high expectations of me. What an embarrassment. *I wanted to crawl into a hole and never come out!!*" [emphasis added]

Feelings of shame involve an acute awareness of one's flawed and unworthy self, a response that often seems out of proportion with the actual severity of the event. For example, Mia, an 18-year-old college student, recalled this shame experience from childhood:

"It is, for some reason, extremely hard to remember. . . . When I was 10, I slept over at a friend's house. His mother came home in the middle of the night and asked if I was cold. I was freezing, but said 'no' to her offer of more blankets. The next day I complained to the friend about how cold I'd been. His mother found out and confronted me with it, and I felt awful—shamefully confused and *unjustified in my existence.*" [emphasis added]

EMPIRICAL STUDIES OF SHAME
VERSUS GUILT EXPERIENCES

In the years since the publication of H. B. Lewis's (1971) book, quite a number of studies have been conducted on the nature of shame and guilt experiences, and the differences between the two. These studies—drawing on both quantitative and qualitative methods—provide impressive empirical support for the distinction proposed by Lewis (Ferguson,

Stegge, & Damhuis, 1990a, 1990b, 1991; Ferguson & Stegge, 1995; Lindsay-Hartz, 1984; Lindsay-Hartz, DeRivera, & Mascolo, 1995; Tangney, 1993b; Tangney et al., 1994; Tangney, Miller, Flicker, & Barlow, 1996; Wicker, Payne, & Morgan, 1983).

For example, in one study (Tangney, 1993b), we asked 65 undergraduate college students to anonymously describe (in writing) a personal shame, guilt, pride, and depression experience. Following each description, they were asked to rate the experience along 22 dimensions using a 7-point scale—dimensions drawn from a review of H. B. Lewis (1971) and Lindsay-Hartz (1984). Of special interest were the participants' ratings of shame and guilt experiences. The results were very consistent with the distinction suggested by Lewis (for details, see Appendix A, Table A.1). Shame and guilt differed in the predicted direction for 17 of the 22 dimensions; the differences were statistically significant for 11 of those 17 dimensions. The students' ratings indicated that their shame experiences were more painful and more difficult to describe than their guilt experiences. Shame was more likely to be accompanied by a sense of being inferior and physically small. These young adults felt they had less control in situations involving shame than in situations involving guilt. And consistent with the painful nature of shame, time was reported to move more slowly in shame than in guilt experiences.

There were also differences in the ways students experienced their relationships with other people when feeling shame as opposed to guilt. When feeling shame, participants were more likely to feel observed by others, and they were also more concerned with others' opinions of the self versus their own self-perception (although, as noted earlier, there was no *objective* difference in how often shame and guilt were experienced alone versus in the presence of other people, nor in how often other people were aware of the participants' behavior). Not surprisingly, people reported a stronger desire to hide from others when feeling shame than when feeling guilt. And when shamed, participants felt more isolated— less as though they belonged—than when experiencing guilt.

In short, these students' ratings of shame and guilt experiences differed along the majority of dimensions postulated by H. B. Lewis (1971),[2] a pattern of findings that is quite striking when one considers that participants described and rated unique personal shame and guilt experiences which spanned a wide range of situations and contexts. Moreover, these results replicate the findings of an earlier investigation by Wicker et al. (1983), and they are remarkably similar to the results of a subsequent study of a larger sample of young adults (Tangney, Miller, et al., 1996).

There was, however, a very notable exception to the support for Lewis's distinction in both studies reported in Tangney (1993b) and Tangney, Miller, et al. (1996). These analyses of phenomenological ratings didn't find the hypothesized difference on the key dimension assessing focus on self versus behavior. As participants recalled each event, they were asked to rate (on a 7-point scale) the degree to which they "blamed my *actions* and behavior" versus "blamed my personality and my *self*." Ratings of this single critical item did not differ across shame and guilt experiences.

We took a close look at this item because it was designed to get to the heart of H. B. Lewis's (1971) distinction between shame and guilt. In hindsight, it appears that this single item may have been an inadequate measure of the dimension of interest—too abstract for college undergraduates with little background in psychology. We conducted some secondary analyses to see if students' ratings of this item made any sense. As it turned out, ratings of this item did not correlate with other rated dimensions in a manner one would expect (Tangney, Miller, et al., 1996). For example, the rating of blaming self versus blaming behavior was uncorrelated with the degree to which participants wished they had *acted* differently, the degree to which they wanted to make amends (both behavior-focused items), and the degree to which they felt *disgusted* with the *self* (a clearly self-focused item). These secondary analyses, together with anecdotal reports from the participants themselves, led us to conclude that the students really didn't understand the distinction we were trying to make.

Subsequently, we adopted an entirely different approach to evaluate Lewis's self versus behavior distinction—an approach that did not require participants themselves to rate and evaluate this rather abstract concept. Instead, we coded participants' counterfactual thinking associated with shame and guilt to explore the self versus behavior distinction (Niedenthal, Tangney, & Gavanski, 1994). Counterfactual thinking involves imagining how past events might have otherwise unfolded if some aspect of the situation or one's actions had been different. For example, having failed an exam, a person might "mentally simulate" alternative scenarios that might have lead to a different outcome (e.g., "If only I had studied more" or "If only I were smarter"). In four independent studies of counterfactual thinking, we found very strong support for H. B. Lewis's (1971) notion that shame and guilt differ in focus on self versus behavior. For example, participants in one study described a personal shame or guilt experience and were then asked to "counterfactualize" the event (e.g., list factors that might have caused the event to end differently, completing the stem "If only . . . "). We then coded the counterfactual responses according to whether aspects of the self, behavior, or situation were "undone." People were observed to more often "undo" aspects of the self in connection with the shame experiences and more often "undo" aspects of their behavior in connection with the guilt experience.

In another study from this series (Niedenthal et al., 1994), we examined whether simply focusing on one's behavior (vs. one's self) might predispose people to experience feelings of guilt (vs. shame). We presented two groups of participants with an identical hypothetical scenario (one that could induce either shame or guilt). One group was then directed to generate statements counterfactualizing the self ("Imagine being a different *type of person*"); the other group was directed to generate statements counterfactualizing the behavior ("Imagine *doing* something different"). Next, participants were asked to rate how much shame and guilt they would experience in such a situation. Results from this study, too, nicely supported H. B. Lewis's (1971) distinction between shame and guilt. Participants who were directed to counterfactualize the self subsequently indicated that they would experience greater shame in a similar situation; participants who counterfactualized behavior indicated that they would experience greater guilt. In all, four independent counterfactual studies, each employing a somewhat different paradigm, support the notion that shame is associated with a focus on the self whereas guilt is associated with a focus on a specific behavior.

Researchers in other labs, too, have found consistent support for Lewis's (1971) conceptualization of shame and guilt. For example, using a very different paradigm, Lindsay-Hartz et al. (1995) interviewed 13 adults at length about personal shame and guilt experiences. They then presented these participants with unlabeled abstract descriptions of various aspects of shame, guilt, anxiety, and depression experiences. Included among these abstract descriptions were statements summarizing shame and guilt "situations," which varied primarily in a focus on the self versus behavior. Participants were able to reliably "match" their own shame and guilt experiences with these abstract descriptions, consistent with Lewis's (1971) distinction between shame and guilt.

In any area of science, it is impressive to see a convergence of results from different investigators employing a range of methodologies. In the decades since the publication of *Shame and Guilt in Neurosis*, Lewis's (1971) conceptualization of shame and guilt has received strong empirical support from qualitative case study analyses (Lewis, 1971; Lindsay-Hartz, 1984; Lindsay-Hartz et al., 1995), content analyses of shame and guilt narratives (Ferguson, Stegge, & Damhuis, 1990a, 1990b; Tangney, 1992; Tangney et al., 1994), participants' quantitative ratings of personal shame and guilt experiences (e.g., Ferguson et al., 1991; Tangney, 1993b; Tangney, Miller, et al., 1996; Wallbott & Scherer, 1995; Wicker et al., 1983), personality and emotional correlates (Gilbert, Pehl, & Allan, 1994), prototype "matching" procedures (Lindsay-Hartz et al., 1995), and analyses of participants' counterfactual thinking (Leith, 1998; Niedenthal et al., 1994). Together, these studies underscore that shame and guilt are distinct emotional experiences that differ substantially along cognitive, affective, and motivational dimensions, as described by Lewis (1971).

SUMMARY AND CONCLUSIONS

Although when asked most people find it difficult to articulate the difference between shame and guilt, empirical research has shown that these are distinct emotions. As it turns out, shame and guilt differ not so much in the content or structure of the situations that engender them, but rather in the manner in which people construe self-relevant negative events. For example, the key difference between shame and guilt does not center merely on a public–private dimension. In fact, there is little empirical support for the commonly held assumption that shame arises from public exposure of some failure or transgression whereas guilt arises from the more private pangs of one's internalized conscience. Rather, there is substantial evidence supporting Lewis's (1971) contention that the fundamental difference between shame and guilt centers on the role of the self. Shame involves fairly global negative evaluations of the self (i.e., "Who *I* am"). Guilt involves a more articulated condemnation of a specific behavior (i.e., "What I *did*"). This difference in focus (self vs. behavior) may seem somewhat subtle at first glance, but it has far-reaching implications for the immediate phenomenological experience of these emotions, for subsequent motivation, and (as we'll see in the remainder of this book) ultimately for behavior. Table 2.1 summarizes some of the key similarities and differences between the experiences of shame and guilt.

TABLE 2.1. Key Similarities and Differences between Shame and Guilt

Features shared by shame and guilt

- Both fall into the class of "moral" emotions.
- Both are "self-conscious," self-referential emotions.
- Both are negatively valanced emotions.
- Both involve internal attributions of one sort or another.
- Both are typically experienced in interpersonal contexts.
- The negative events that give rise to shame and guilt are highly similar (frequently involving moral failures or transgressions).

Key dimensions on which shame and guilt differ

	Shame	Guilt
Focus of evaluation	Global self: "*I* did that horrible thing"	Specific behavior: "I *did* that horrible *thing*"
Degree of distress	Generally more painful than guilt	Generally less painful than shame
Phenomenological experience	Shrinking, feeling small, feeling worthless, powerless	Tension, remorse, regret
Operation of "self"	Self "split" into observing and observed "selves"	Unified self intact
Impact on "self"	Self impaired by global devaluation	Self unimpaired by global devaluation
Concern vis-à-vis the "other"	Concern with others' evaluation of self	Concern with one's effect on others
Counterfactual processes	Mentally undoing some aspect of the self	Mentally undoing some aspect of behavior
Motivational features	Desire to hide, escape, or strike back	Desire to confess, apologize, or repair

NOTES

1. Throughout the book, we use pseudonyms to protect the anonymity of research participants, but these are actual quotes from our studies.
2. Two dimensions yielded reliable differences counter to H. B. Lewis's (1971) distinction. Participants indicated that, in the shame experiences, they were more likely to feel they had violated a moral standard and more likely to wish they had acted differently. In contrast, Lewis (1971) anticipated that guilt would be more consistently tied to violations of moral standards and more clearly focused on regrets of action (vs. negative evaluations of the global self). It seems likely that the contradictory findings stem in part from the greater aversiveness of shame experiences. (Shame events were rated as substantially more painful than guilt events.) In rating the latter dimension, participants may have focused not on the question of actions, but rather on whether they wished something about the situation, more generally, to be different. Regarding the violation of moral standards, respondents may have retrospectively interpreted the shame-eliciting transgression as more severe once they construed the "immoral" behavior as an even more serious reflection of an "immoral" self.

Chapter 3

ASSESSING SHAME AND GUILT

Are feelings of shame and guilt equally likely to foster moral behavior? Are guilt-prone people more likely to experience psychological symptoms? What kind? And are these different for shame-prone individuals? In what ways do feelings of shame and guilt protect or enhance our interpersonal relationships? In what ways can shame and guilt hinder or harm our relationships with others? Where does the capacity for shame and guilt come from? Is there really such a thing as a guilt-inducing mother? Is that a good or bad thing? More generally, how can parents help foster the development of an adaptive moral emotional style in their children?

To answer these questions in any systematic fashion, researchers need a way to measure shame and guilt. But, as it turns out, the measurement of these emotions poses a real challenge. Shame and guilt are internal affective states that are difficult, if not impossible, to assess directly. For example, unlike most of the "primary" emotions (e.g., anger, sadness, joy), shame and guilt do not involve clearly definable, codable facial expressions (Izard, 1977). There is no clear-cut "guilt" expression, nor a readily recognizable "shame" expression.

When we look instead to people's words—their verbal reports of their feelings—other problems arise. Most laypersons (and many psychologists) are rather unclear about the distinction between shame and guilt. So if you ask a person, "How much are you feeling guilt right now?" or "In general, do you feel guilt infrequently, occasionally, often, or very often?" that person's answers may tell you something about his or her feelings of guilt, shame, or both. And if there is a single most important "take-home message" from this book, it is that making a clear distinction between shame and guilt is critically important in both our theoretical formulations and in our measures.

The past 10 years or so have seen a dramatic increase in empirical studies of shame and guilt, in large part due to the recent development of a number of new measures. In this chapter, we review the range of approaches that have been developed for measuring shame and guilt (both as states and as dispositions), commenting on their relative strengths and weaknesses. In addition, because our measures of shame and guilt, the Tests of Self-Conscious Affect (TOSCA), were used in many of the studies referenced in the remainder of this book, we describe in some detail the development of TOSCA for adults, TOSCA-A for adolescents, and TOSCA-C for children, and their precursors, the Self-Conscious Affect and Attribution Inventories (SCAAI). (Copies of the most recent TOSCA measures can be found in Appendix B.)

In evaluating the relative strengths and weaknesses of various measurement strategies, two related issues need to be considered: First, what *definitions* of shame and guilt underlie a given measure? To what degree was the development of the measure guided by empirically supported definitions and distinctions between shame and guilt? Second, how well does the *operationalization* of shame and guilt map on to these definitions? Here, it is important to consider both the form and the content of the measure.

Measures of shame and guilt can be classified into two broad categories: (1) those which assess emotional *states* (e.g., feelings of shame and guilt in the moment), and (2) those which assess emotional traits or *dispositions* (e.g., shame-proneness and guilt-proneness). Far more effort has been devoted to the development of dispositional measures, so we begin with a review of these assessment methods.

DISPOSITIONAL MEASURES:
SHAME-PRONENESS AND GUILT-PRONENESS

The notion underlying dispositional measures is that, although most people have a capacity to experience both emotions at various points in their lives, there are individual differences in the degree to which people are prone to experience shame and/or guilt across a range of situations involving failures or transgressions.

Measures Assessing Only One of the Two Dispositions

A number of scales, particularly earlier measures of these constructs, have been developed that assess guilt-proneness without a consideration of shame-proneness (Buss & Durkee, 1957; Klass, 1987; Kubany, et al., 1996; Kugler & Jones, 1992; Mosher, 1966; O'Connor, Berry, Weiss, Bushi, & Sampson, 1997; Otterbacher & Munz, 1973; Zahn-Waxler, Kochanska, Krupnick, & Mayfield, 1988), or vice versa (Cook, 1989). As described in greater detail in Table 3.1, these measures draw on a range of different formats: selection of a single adjective, ratings of descriptive statements, forced-choice alternatives, ratings of likely emotional responses to specific situations, and qualitative analysis of narrative responses to specific situations.

Problems Distinguishing between Shame and Guilt

One problem with many of these measures, particularly those assessing guilt-proneness only, is that they have not taken into account the difference between shame and guilt. As a result, they end up assessing (and confounding) the two emotions and so are of little use in examining the differential roles of shame and guilt in various aspects of psychological and social functioning. For example, the Buss–Durkee Guilt Scale (Buss & Durkee, 1957) includes such items as "I sometimes have bad thoughts which make me feel ashamed of myself" and "I often feel that I have not lived the right kind of life." The Mosher Forced-Choice Guilt Inventory (Mosher, 1966) includes such items as "I detest myself for . . . (a) my sins and failures, vs. (b) not having more exciting sexual experiences" and "If I felt like murdering someone . . . (a) I would be ashamed of myself, vs. (b) I would try to commit the perfect crime." Three of the most heavily weighted guilt adjectives on the G-Trait scale of the Perceived Guilt Index (PGI; Otterbacher & Munz, 1973) are "Disgraceful," "Degraded," and "Marred," items which, if anything, more clearly suggest experiences of shame than guilt. Zahn-Waxler et al. (1988) include as criteria for a guilt response any indication that the child was at fault or *blamed the self* (e.g., "She feels like a bad girl"). Klass's (1987) Situational Guilt Scale most blatantly confounds shame and guilt, summing respondents' ratings of how much they would feel "regretful," "disap-

TABLE 3.1. Measures Assessing Either Guilt-Proneness or Shame-Proneness

Measures assessing guilt-proneness but not shame-proneness

Adult measures

- Forced-Choice Guilt Inventory (FCGI; Mosher, 1966). This measure is composed of 79 incomplete sentence stems, each followed by two completions. People are "forced to make a choice" between the two completions. The FCGI yields three subscales: Hostility–Guilt (29 items), Sex–Guilt (28 items), and Morality–Conscience (22 items).

- Guilt Inventory (Kugler & Jones, 1992). This measure includes a Trait Guilt Scale composed of 20 items (e.g., "Guilt and remorse have been a part of my life for as long as I can recall"). People rate how well each item describes themselves on a 5-point scale.

- Hostility–Guilt Inventory (Buss & Durkee, 1957). The Buss–Durkee Inventory includes a 9-item Guilt Scale. People indicate whether they agree or disagree with 9 descriptive statements (e.g., "I am concerned about being forgiven for my sins").

- Interpersonal Guilt Questionnaire–45 (IGQ-45; O'Connor et al., 1997) is a 45-item measure yielding four subscales: Survivor Guilt, Separation/Disloyalty Guilt, Omnipotent Responsibility Guilt, and Self-Hate Guilt.

- Perceived Guilt Index (PGI; Otterbacher & Munz, 1973). The G-Trait scale of the PGI is essentially a single-item measure. People are asked to select one adjective from a list of 11 adjectives (varying in level of guilt) that best describes how they "normally feel."

- Situational Guilt Scale (Klass, 1987). On this measure, people rate their likely emotional reactions to 22 specific situations presumed to induce guilt.

- Trauma-Related Guilt Inventory (TRGI; Kubany et al., 1996) is a 32-item measure that yields scales assessing Global Guilt (4 items), Distress (6 items), and Guilt Cognitions (22 items). The Guilt Cognitions scale can be broken down into three subscales assessing Hindsight–Bias/Responsibility, Wrongdoing, and Lack of Justification.

Child measure

- Children's Interpretations of Interpersonal Distress and Conflict (CIIDC; Zahn-Waxler et al., 1988). Guilt scores can be derived by coding children's responses to this projective measure. Children are presented with photographs of four ambiguous situations (e.g., a child watching an adult female—described as angry—leaving a room) and asked to describe the situation, characters' feelings, etc. (see also Zahn-Waxler, Kochanska, Krupnick, & McKnew, 1990).

Measures assessing shame-proneness but not guilt-proneness

Adult measures

- Internalized Shame Scale (ISS; Cook, 1989). The most recent version of the ISS is composed of 24 items (with 6 items from the Rosenberg Self-Esteem scale as fillers), each rated on a 5-point scale. Cook (1988) defines "internalized shame" as an "enduring, chronic shame that has become internalized as part of one's identity and which can be most succinctly characterized as a deep sense of inferiority, inadequacy, or deficiency."

- Shame Interview assessing shame about one's body (B. Andrews, 1995) and feelings of shame in response to more general situations (B. Andrews & Hunter, 1997) distinguishing between "characterological" and "behavioral" shame.

- Experience of Shame Scale (B. Andrews, Qian, & Valentine, in press) is a 25-item questionnaire based on B. Andrews and Hunter's (1997) interview, yielding measures of bodily shame, characterological shame, and behavioral shame.

pointed in myself," "guilty," and "ashamed" when faced with each of 22 specific situations to calculate a total "guilt" score. Among these measures, Kugler and Jones's (1992) Trait Guilt Scale is the only one which involved some explicit effort to take into account the distinction between shame and guilt. These authors made a deliberate attempt to screen out shame items, and seem to have been successful in doing so with only a few exceptions (e.g., "Frequently, I just hate myself for something I have done").

Researchers who use measures that confound shame and guilt run the risk of obtaining quite misleading results. Much of the research summarized in the remainder of this book shows that when shame-proneness and guilt-proneness are assessed as distinct constructs, they show very different relationships to many aspects of psychological adjustment and social behavior, including psychological symptoms, narcissism, sociopathy, interpersonal empathy, anger, aggression, constructive anger management strategies, and aspects of interpersonal perception (Brodie, 1995; Gramzow & Tangney, 1992; Petersen, Barlow, & Tangney, 1995; Sanftner, Barlow, Marschall, & Tangney, 1995; Tangney, 1991, 1994, 1995a, 1995b, 1995c; Tangney, Burggraf, & Wagner, 1995; Tangney, Wagner, Barlow, Marschall, & Gramzow, 1996; Tangney, Wagner, Fletcher, & Gramzow, 1992; Tangney, Wagner, & Gramzow, 1992). It is not unusual to find that the correlations of shame-proneness and guilt-proneness with some other construct of interest are marked by differences not just in magnitude but also in *direction* or "sign." So when a researcher uses a "guilt" measure that unwittingly includes elements of shame, he or she may observe negligible correlations and erroneously conclude that these emotions are irrelevant to the variable of interest, when in fact two noteworthy but opposing relationships have essentially canceled one another out!

Problems Distinguishing between Guilt and Moral Standards

In addition to the distinction between shame and guilt, several other distinctions should be considered when researchers are evaluating the discriminant validity of measures of shame and/or guilt.[1] Some measures confound proneness to guilt with moral standards or other related attitudes and beliefs. This conceptual ambiguity is perhaps most evident in the Mosher Forced-Choice Guilt Inventory (Mosher, 1966), which includes such items as "One should not . . . (a) knowingly sin, vs. (b) try to follow absolutes" (Morality–Conscience item), "Sex relations before marriage . . . (a) ruin many a happy couple, vs. (b) are good in my opinion" (Sex–Guilt item), and "Capital punishment . . . (a) should be abolished, vs. (b) is a necessity" (Hostility–Guilt item). These kinds of items stray rather far afield from feelings of guilt, focusing instead on morally relevant standards and beliefs.

Although feelings of guilt generally arise from some failure or violation of moral standards, proneness to guilt (an *affective disposition*) is conceptually distinct from moral standards (a *set of values*). Proneness to guilt is an emotional style—a tendency to experience guilt (as opposed to something else) in response to one's failures or transgressions. Moral standards are the set of *beliefs* against which people judge their behavior. It's not clear why the degree to which an individual is guilt-prone would be directly tied to the *content* of that individual's standards for moral conduct. For example, people with relatively "unconventional" moral standards may be just as likely to evaluate their own moral violations negatively (self-defined) as people who endorse more mainstream standards of conduct.

Moreover, there's no reason to expect a one-to-one correspondence between the "stringency" of a person's moral standards and the degree to which he or she is prone to guilt. That is, even among people with "high" moral standards (conventional or otherwise), some may be relatively prone to guilt whereas others may not. First, people vary in the degree to which they actually transgress—in the opportunities they create for themselves to experience guilt. Some people hold high moral standards *and* live exemplary lives; others do not. Second, and more important, people vary in the degree to which they are willing or able to acknowledge their transgressions. For example, George enthusiastically subscribes to a stringent code of moral conduct (in the abstract), but at the same time he has an elaborate system of defenses and rationalizations vis-à-vis his own behavior, thus protecting himself from daily experiences of guilt. No matter what, George never does wrong! It's always the other guy! George's neighbor Ronald shares the same values and moral beliefs, but in sharp contrast Ronald is quick to admit when he himself has trangressed or erred. For him, there's no double standard. He evaluates himself as stringently as he evaluates others. So George and Ronald share the same moral standards, but psychologists might view Ronald (being less defensive) as more prone to guilt. In this regard, some findings involving Kugler and Jones's (1992) Guilt Inventory are especially noteworthy. Unlike the Mosher Force-Choice Guilt Inventory, Kugler and Jones's (1992) Guilt Inventory explicitly distinguishes between "Trait Guilt" and "Moral Standards." In an initial set of validation studies, Kugler and Jones (1992) reported essentially no relationship between these two subscales, further underscoring the importance of distinguishing between "moral affect" and "moral standards," both conceptually and methodologically.

Problems Distinguishing between Shame and Self-Esteem

Issues of discriminant validity are important when researchers are considering measures of shame as well as guilt. Here, the distinction between shame and self-esteem warrants particular attention. Cook's (1989) Internalized Shame Scale (ISS) perhaps most clearly illustrates this ambiguity. Cook (1988) has defined "internalized shame" as an "enduring, chronic shame that has become internalized as part of one's identity and which can be most succinctly characterized as a deep sense of inferiority, inadequacy, or deficiency" (p. 9). A key question is how this sort of "internalized shame" differs from low self-esteem. Cook (1988) attempted to distinguish theoretically between the two constructs, noting that whereas internalized shame is an extremely painful affect experienced around a basic sense of inferiority, negative self-esteem is a "less dynamic" concept centering on self-description or self rating. The haziness of this distinction is reflected in the content of the ISS shame items, many of which clearly tap self-esteem issues (e.g., "I feel like I am never quite good enough," "Compared to other people, I feel like I somehow never measure up," and "I see myself striving for perfection only to continually fall short"). Not surprisingly, the ISS correlates very highly with measures of self-esteem. Earlier versions of the ISS correlated −.81 to −.88 with the Coopersmith (1967) and M. Rosenberg (1965) self-esteem scales (Cook, 1988). Similarly, Cook (1991) reported that the more recent version of the ISS correlates substantially with measures of self-esteem (−.52 to −.79). Notably, in those studies that showed the more modest correlations, the relationship of self-esteem scales (e.g., the Coopersmith, 1967, and the Tennessee Self-Concept Scale, Fitts, 1965) to Cook's (ISS) Shame scale (−.52 and −.66, respectively) were virtually identical to those with Cook's (ISS) Self-Esteem scale (drawing on Rosenberg items), again raising the question of discriminant validity.

One can certainly imagine how proneness to shame might contribute to problems with self-esteem (and vice versa), but these are nonetheless distinct constructs. Global self-esteem is a stable trait involving a person's general evaluation of the self, largely independent of specific situations. Theoretical definitions vary in their emphasis on affective and cognitive components. But self-esteem is essentially a *self*-evaluative construct. Shame is an emotion—an affective state. The corresponding trait or disposition is shame-proneness—a tendency to experience the emotion shame (as opposed to, say, indifference or guilt) in response to specific negative events. (See Chapter 4 for a more extended discussion of the distinction between shame and self-esteem.) The ISS—as well as the theoretical work on which it was apparently based (Kaufman, 1985, 1989)—blurs this distinction. This is unfortunate because, in effect, it rules out the possibility of exploring the functional links between self-esteem and shame (or shame-proneness)—or the differential relationship of these variables to other aspects of personality and adjustment.

Rather than rewriting some 50 years of literature on self-esteem by reconceptualizing self-esteem as internalized shame, we think it may be more useful to carefully delineate this distinction—in both theory and assessment method.

Measures Assessing (and Distinguishing between) Shame-Proneness and Guilt-Proneness

Since the appearance of H. B. Lewis's (1971) landmark *Shame and Guilt in Neurosis*, researchers have become increasingly aware of the importance of distinguishing between shame and guilt. As a result, a number of assessment techniques have been developed which attempt to assess dispositional guilt distinct from dispositional shame, and vice versa. (See Table 3.2.) Again, these measures vary substantially in structure or format. Here, it is important to examine carefully the theoretical assumptions that have shaped each approach because the selection of a particular measurement format is not simply a matter of taste. Whether implicit or explicit, quite different conceptual distinctions underlie these various approaches to assessing shame-prone and guilt-prone styles.

Shame- versus Guilt-Inducing Situations

One approach is to assess the degree to which respondents would react to a range of "shame-inducing" versus "guilt-inducing" situations. This approach was first introduced by Perlman (1958), who devised a measure composed of 26 situations presumably likely to induce shame and 26 situations presumably likely to induce guilt. A respondent is asked

TABLE 3.2. Measures Assessing both Shame-Proneness and Guilt-Proneness

Shame- versus guilt-inducing situations

Several measures assess reactions to presumably distinct "shame-inducing" versus "guilt-inducing" situations (Perlman, 1958; Beall, 1972; Johnson et al., 1987; Cheek & Hogan, 1983).

- Anxiety Attitude Survey (AAS; Perlman, 1958). This measure is composed of 26 situations presumably likely to induce shame and 26 situations presumably likely to induce guilt. Respondents rate on a 9-point scale how anxious "most people would be were this to happen to them." Ratings for "shame-inducing" versus "guilt-inducing" situations are aggregated to create indices of shame-proneness and guilt-proneness, respectively.

- Beall Shame–Guilt Test (Beall, 1972). Respondents rate how much they themselves would be "upset" by a series of presumably shame- and guilt-inducing situations (e.g., "You find a lost wallet. It has only five dollars. You take the money and then turn the wallet in." and "You feel a nagging worry that you are not doing what you should do to help solve social problems."). Ratings for "shame-inducing" versus "guilt-inducing" situations are aggregated to create indices of shame-proneness and guilt-proneness, respectively.

- Measure of Susceptibility to Guilt and Shame (Cheek & Hogan, 1983). This measure is composed of 5 situations presumably likely to induce shame and 5 situations presumably likely to induce guilt. Respondents rate on a 5-point scale "the guilt or shame you would feel in each situation." Ratings for "shame-inducing" versus "guilt-inducing" situations are aggregated to create indices of shame-proneness and guilt-proneness, respectively.

- Dimensions of Conscience Questionnaire (DCQ; Johnson et al., 1987). This measure is an abbreviated 28-item version of a much longer (121 item) instrument developed by Johnson and Noel (1970). Respondents rate on a 7-point scale "how badly they would feel after committing" 13 "shame-inducing" and 15 "guilt-inducing" situations. Ratings are aggregated to create indices of shame-proneness and guilt-proneness, respectively.

Global adjective checklists

- Revised Shame–Guilt Scale (RSGS; Hoblitzelle, 1987) consists of 16 shame adjectives and 20 guilt adjectives. Respondents use a 5-point scale to rate how well each adjective describes the self.

- Personal Feelings Questionnaire (PFQ; Harder & Lewis, 1987). Respondents are presented with a list of 5 shame and 3 guilt-related affective descriptors and asked to rate the frequency with which they experience such feelings.

- Personal Feelings Questionnaire–2 (PFQ-2; Harder et al., 1992). An expansion of the PFQ consisting of 10 shame- and 6 guilt-related affective descriptors (e.g., for guilt, "intense guilt," "regret," "remorse," "worry about hurting or injuring another"; for shame, "embarrassment," "feeling ridiculous," "feeling childish," "feeling disgusting to others").

Scenario-based measures

Measures for adults

- Self-Conscious Affect and Attribution Inventory (SCAAI; Tangney et al., 1988) is the forerunner of the TOSCA measures; it was developed for use with college

TABLE 3.2. (*continued*)

students. The SCAAI is composed of 13 situations commonly experienced by college students, each followed by several possible responses. Across the various scenarios, the responses capture affective, cognitive, and behavioral features associated with shame and guilt. Also included are items assessing externalization of blame, detachment/unconcern, alpha pride (pride in self), and beta pride (pride in behavior).

- Test of Self-Conscious Affect (TOSCA; Tangney et al., 1989) was modeled after the SCAAI. The TOSCA also consists of a series of brief scenarios (10 negative and 5 positive) and associated responses, yielding indices of Shame, Guilt, Externalization, Detachment/Unconcern, Alpha Pride, and Beta Pride subscales. This entirely new set of scenarios was drawn from written accounts of personal shame, guilt, and pride experiences provided by a sample of several hundred college students and noncollege adults. The new responses were drawn from a much larger pool of affective, cognitive, and behavioral responses provided by a second sample of noncollege adults, thus enhancing the ecological validity of the measure. The measure was developed for adults of all ages, not specifically college students.

- Test of Self-Conscious Affect–2 (TOSCA-2; Tangney, Ferguson, et al., 1996) augmented the TOSCA with a new subscale aimed at tapping a chronic, ruminative, unresolved type of guilt—the Maladaptive Guilt scale. In creating the TOSCA-2, we also added two new scenarios and deleted one original scenario. Subsequent analyses indicated problems with the discriminant validity of the Maladaptive Guilt scale vis-à-vis shame.

- Test of Self-Conscious Affect–3 (TOSCA-3; Tangney et al., 2000), the most recent version of our adult measure, retains the 16 scenarios from the TOSCA-2 but eliminates the Maladaptive Guilt scale owing to problems with discriminant validity. In addition, the TOSCA-3 includes the option of a shorter 10-scenario version (dropping positive scenarios).

- Test of Self-Conscious Affect–SD (TOSCA-SD; Hanson & Tangney, 1995) is a 10-scenario version of the TOSCA modifed for use with "socially deviant" populations, especially incarcerated individuals.

Measures for children and adolescents

- Child Attribution and Reaction Survey—Child Version (C-CARS; Stegge & Ferguson, 1990) is a "down-aged" version of the TOSCA-C composed of 8 scenarios appropriate for children as young as 5 years.

- Self-Conscious Affect and Attribution Inventory for Children (SCAAI-C; Burggraf & Tangney, 1989), the forerunner of the TOSCA-C, was modeled after the SCAAI for adults. Like the SCAAI, it is composed of a series of common age-appropriate situations, each followed by several possible responses. To accommodate this age group, illustrations were added to help the children keep the scenarios in mind while working through the responses, and 5-point numerically anchored Likert scales were replaced with a string of 5 circles graded in size. Like the SCAAI, the SCAAI-C yields Shame, Guilt, Externalization of Blame, Detachment/Unconcern, Alpha Pride (pride in self), and Beta Pride (pride in behavior) subscales.

- Test of Self-Conscious Affect for Children (TOSCA-C; Tangney et al., 1990) was modeled after the SCAAI-C. The TOSCA-C, appropriate for children ages 8–12, consists of a series of brief scenarios (10 negative and 5 positive) and associated responses, yielding indices of Shame, Guilt, Externalization of Blame, Detachment/ Unconcern, Alpha Pride, and Beta Pride subscales. This entirely new set of scenarios

(*continued*)

TABLE 3.2. (*continued*)

was drawn from written accounts of personal shame, guilt, and pride experiences provided by a diverse sample of over 100 elementary school children. The new responses were drawn from a much larger pool of affective, cognitive, and behavioral responses provided by a second sample of elementary-school-age children.

• Test of Self-Conscious Affect for Adolescents (TOSCA-A; Tangney, Wagner, Gavlas, & Gramzow, 1991a) is composed of 15 scenarios and associated responses, yielding indices of Shame, Guilt, Externalization of Blame, Detachment/Unconcern, Alpha Pride, and Beta Pride subscales. TOSCA-A scenarios and responses were drawn from the TOSCA and TOSCA-C; based on pilot work with several hundred adolescents, items were rewritten and the format was revised to yield an age-appropriate measure for adolescents.

Measures assessing state shame and/or guilt

• Differential Emotions Scale (DES; Izard, 1977). Various forms of the DES exist, some relying on single-word descriptors of key emotions (e.g., guilt, shyness, sadness) and others drawing on clusters of closely related emotion words to describe each key emotion (e.g., for guilt: repentant, guilty, blameworthy), each rated on a 5-point scale in reference to the respondent's current feeling state. Mosher and White (1981) modified the DES to provide separate shame, embarrassment, and shyness clusters.

• Experiential Shame Scale (ESS; Turner, 1998) is composed of 9 semantic differential items assessing physical, emotional, and social markers of shame experiences "in the moment." Terms such as "shame," "embarrassment," and "humiliation" are not used. The ESS was developed as an implicit ("opaque") measure of shame to circumvent defensive responding.

• State Guilt Scale (Kugler & Jones, 1992), part of the Guilt Inventory, is composed of 10 items such as "I have recently done something that I deeply regret." Like many dispositional measures that do not explicitly attempt to assess and distinguish between shame and guilt, some of the items seem likely to tap shame experiences (e.g., "Lately, it hasn't been easy being me." and "Lately, I have felt good about myself and what I have done.") as well as guilt experiences.

• State Shame and Guilt Scale (SSGS; Marschall et al., 1994) is composed of brief phenomenological descriptions of shame (5 items, e.g., "I feel humiliated, disgraced," "I want to sink into the floor and disappear") and guilt (5 items, e.g., "I feel remorse, regret," "I cannot stop thinking about something bad I have done") experiences, each rated on a 5-point scale.

Note. See Table 3.3 for pros and cons.

to rate on a 9-point scale how "anxious he [*sic*] feels most people would be were this to happen to them" (p. 753). Ratings for "shame-inducing" versus "guilt-inducing" situations are aggregated to create indices of shame-proneness and guilt-proneness, respectively. A similar approach has been taken by Beall (1972, cited in R. L. Smith, 1972, and Crouppen, 1976), Johnson et al. (1987), and Cheek and Hogan (1983). On the Beall Shame–Guilt Test, for example, respondents rate how much they themselves would be "upset" by a series of presumably shame- and guilt-inducing situations (e.g., "You find a lost wallet. It has only five dollars. You take the money and then turn the wallet in" and "You feel a nagging worry that you are not doing what you should do to help solve social problems"). The critical assumption underlying each of these measures is that there are significant differences in the types of situations that elicit shame and guilt (i.e., that shame and guilt are distinguished precisely by differences in the content of eliciting situations). But as discussed in Chapter 2, there is much theoretical and empirical work challenging this notion. So the basic premise of these measures is, at best, questionable. Researchers would be well advised to carefully examine the assumptions underlying such measures before selecting this type of assessment.

Global Adjective Checklists

A second approach draws on a checklist of shame- and guilt-related adjectives. People are asked to make global ratings of how well each adjective describes the self. For example, Hoblitzelle's (1987a, 1987b) Revised Shame–Guilt Scale (RSGS; adapted from Gioiella's [1981], Shame/Guilt Scale) consists of 16 shame adjectives (e.g., mortified, humiliated, embarrassed) and 20 guilt adjectives (e.g., unethical, liable, culpable). A respondent is asked to rate the degree to which each adjective describes him- or herself (e.g., on a 5-point scale). Harder and colleagues (Harder & Lewis, 1987; Harder, Cutler, & Rockart, 1992) have developed the Personal Feelings Questionnaire (PFQ) and the revised PFQ-2. In these measures, respondents are presented with a list of shame- and guilt-related affective descriptors (e.g., for guilt, "intense guilt," "regret," "remorse," "worry about hurting or injuring another"; for shame, "embarrassment," "feeling ridiculous," "feeling childish," "feeling disgusting to others") and asked to rate the frequency with which they experience such feelings. The PFQ is composed of 5 shame items and 3 guilt items. The PFQ-2 is composed of 10 shame items and 6 guilt items.

Advantages and Limitations. These measures certainly have high face validity—they look as though they ought to measure shame and guilt. Moreover, they are easy to administer. But several problems arise with this approach. From a practical standpoint, extended adjective checklists like the RSGS require very advanced verbal skills. In our own research, we have found that most college students are unfamiliar with at least some of the words on the RSGS. (One of us, June Tangney, had to look some of them up herself, just to be sure.) This is less a problem with the PFQ measures, which involve less sophisticated vocabulary. However, the PFQ and the PFQ-2 rely heavily on respondents' ability to distinguish between the terms "shame" and "guilt" in an abstract context. In the case of the PFQ, two of the three guilt items make use of the term "guilt" (e.g., "intense guilt"); similarly two of the six PFQ-2 items center on the term "guilt" (e.g., "mild guilt" and "intense guilt"). Although such items have good face validity, there is reason to question whether respondents are able to rate their frequency of guilt experiences as conceptually independent of shame experiences using this method. Research has shown that even well-educated adults have difficulty providing meaningful definitions of shame and guilt in the abstract (Lindsay-Hartz, 1984; Tangney, 1989). Moreover, H. B. Lewis (1971) has noted that when both shame and guilt are evoked by the same event, the two states tend to fuse with each other, and are then typically labeled "guilt." In fact, many people use the term "guilt" to refer to both experiences, more generally. So it seems likely that in rating several key PFQ/PFQ-2 guilt items, respondents are apt to report on a generalized tendency to experience negative self-directed affect (e.g., both guilt and shame)—again raising concerns about discriminant validity.

The difficulties with the adjective checklist approach do not end there. As mentioned earlier, when evaluating the validity of any operationalization of shame and guilt, it is important to consider the form as well as the content of the measure at hand. The most problematic aspect of the global adjective approach, in our view, is that it essentially poses respondents with a shame-like task—that of making global ratings about the self (or the self's general affective state) in the absence of any specific situational context (Tangney et al., 1995; Tangney, 1995a, 1995b, 1996). This is not so much a problem for the assessment of shame, which involves rather global negative assessments of the entire self. But it is a serious problem when attempting to assess a dispositional tendency to experience guilt—guilt about specific behaviors, somewhat apart from the global self.

Scenario-Based Measures

A third method for assessing shame-proneness and guilt-proneness is the scenario-based approach (Burggraf & Tangney, 1989; Stegge &

Ferguson, 1990; Tangney, Burggraf, Hamme, & Domingos, 1988; Tangney, Wagner, Burggraf, Gramzow, & Fletcher, 1990; Tangney, Wagner, Gavlas, & Gramzow, 1991a, 1991b; Tangney, Wagner, & Gramzow, 1989; Tangney, 1990). In these measures, respondents are presented with a series of specific common day-to-day situations (e.g., "You make a big mistake on an important project at work. People were depending on you and your boss criticizes you."). Each scenario is followed by responses representing brief phenomenological descriptions of shame and guilt with respect to the specific context (e.g., for shame, "You would feel like you wanted to hide"; for guilt, "You would think 'I should have recognized the problem and done a better job.' "). Across the various scenarios, the responses capture affective, cognitive, and behavioral features associated with shame and guilt, respectively (as described in the theoretical, phenomenological, and empirical literature) without relying on the terms "shame" and "guilt" that may confuse laypersons. It should be noted that these measures are not forced-choice. Respondents are asked to rate, on a 5-point scale, their likelihood of responding in each manner indicated. This approach allows for the possibility that some respondents may experience both shame and guilt in connection with a given situation.

Although these scenario-based measures bear a superficial resemblance to the "shame-vs.-guilt situation" measures described earlier, there are important and fundamental differences between the structures of the two sets of measures and between the theoretical assumptions that informed the measures. The "shame-vs.-guilt situation" measures (Perlman, 1958; Beall, 1972; Johnson et al., 1987; Cheek & Hogan, 1983) rest on the dubious assumption that different kinds of situations elicit shame and guilt, respectively. In sharp contrast, the format of these more recent scenario-based measures explicitly allows for the possibility that a given situation can elicit feelings of shame or guilt, or both. The distinction here is not in the content of the situation but in the phenomenological reaction of the respondent.

Advantages of Scenario-Based Measures. There are several key advantages to this scenario-based approach. Most important, the structure of scenario-based measures is more conceptually consistent with current notions of guilt. Guilt is an emotion that stems from a negative evaluation of specific behaviors, embedded in local contexts. So this situation-specific approach seems uniquely well suited for assessing guilt. It circumvents the global nature of adjective rating scales that are devoid of specific contexts and behaviors, and thus more representative of shame. Instead, scenario-based measures provide a vehicle for assessing tendencies to experience guilt about specific behaviors, distinct from shame about the self.

A second advantage of the scenario-based approach is that it is composed of situation-specific phenomenological descriptions of shame and guilt, rather than relying on respondents' ability to distinguish between the terms "shame" and "guilt" in the abstract. In fact, the SCAAI and TOSCA measures do not use the terms "shame" and "guilt" at all.

Third, this approach seems less likely to arouse defensive response biases than adjective checklist-type measures. In fact, Harder and Lewis (1987) raised concerns that by asking participants to provide global self-reports of shame reactions (e.g., directly asking subjects to rate the frequency or degree to which they experience shame), the PFQ may invite a defensive denial on the part of some participants. This is not a minor concern, for as H. B. Lewis (1971) and others have noted, a fair proportion of individuals routinely repress or deny shame experiences and some people may not even recognize the shame experience as such. Scenario-based measures may, in part, circumvent people's defensiveness because they are asked to rate phenomenological descriptions of shame and guilt experiences with respect to specific situations, rather than being asked to acknowledge global tendencies to experience SHAME and GUILT bluntly. Perhaps more than most other emotion words, "shame" and "guilt" are emotionally charged words for many individuals. Respondents may be more willing to acknowledge "feeling small . . . like a rat" (shame) or "thinking it over several times, wondering if you could have avoided it" (guilt) in reference to a particular situation, rather than in general feeling "disgusting to others" or feeling "intense guilt" frequently or continuously.

Finally, scenario-based measures can be more easily adapted for use with younger participants. In fact, in addition to the 15-scenario TOSCA (Tangney et al., 1989), and its forerunner, the 13-scenario SCAAI (Tangney et al., 1988; Tangney, 1990), we have developed a 15-scenario TOSCA-A for adolescents (Tangney, Wagner, Gavlas, & Gramzow, 1991a) and a 15-scenario TOSCA-C for children ages 8–12 (Tangney, Wagner, Burggraf, Gramzow, & Fletcher, 1990), modeled after the SCAAI-C for children (Burggraf & Tangney, 1989). Stegge and Ferguson (1990) have also developed a down-aged version of the TOSCA-C, the 8-scenario Child Attribution and Reaction Survey—

Child Version (C-CARS) appropriate for children as young as 5 years. Each of these measures presents respondents with a range of age-appropriate situations (sampling from home, work/school, peer groups, and other domains) that are likely to elicit shame and/or guilt. In addition to shame and guilt items, these measures include responses tapping externalization of blame, detachment/unconcern, and—for a subset of ostensibly positive situations—pride in self and pride in behavior.

Limitations of Scenario-Based Measures. These scenario-based measures are not without drawbacks and limitations. First, regarding *reliability*, one of the first steps in evaluating a measurement scale involves looking at how well the items covary, or "hang together." If each of the 15 items on a shame scale is designed to assess shame, a high shame-prone person should endorse all the items in a similar manner. Similarly, low shame-prone individuals should rate all shame items relatively low. The result of such consistent response patterns is a scale with high internal consistency—one of the marks of a psychometrically sound scale. In general, scenario-based measures yield somewhat lower internal consistency estimates of reliability than do the adjective checklist measures.[2] Note, however, that coefficient alpha tends to underestimate reliability in scenario-based measures because of the situation variance introduced by this scenario approach. In other words, the items of a given scale share common variance due to the psychological construct of interest, but each item also includes unique variance associated with its own scenario. This results in an underestimate of reliability. In this context, alpha estimates of internal consistency for the TOSCA scales are reasonably high for a scenario-based measure. Not surprisingly, test–retest reliabilities for these scenario-based measures tend to be higher. For example, in a study of undergraduates, stabilities over a 3- to 5-week period were .85 and .74 for the TOSCA Shame and Guilt scales, respectively (Tangney, Wagner, Fletcher, & Gramzow, 1992), which is comparable to those reported for the PFQ (Harder & Lewis, 1987).

A second limitation has to do with the inevitable *constraints on the range of shame- and guilt-inducing situations* included in these measures. In constructing the SCAAI and TOSCA measures, we made an explicit attempt to include scenarios from diverse settings (e.g., home, work/school, peer groups, and other domains) focusing on diverse behaviors (e.g., missing an appointment, breaking something, accidentally hitting someone, hurting another person's feelings, procrastinating, failing a test). Nonetheless, each measure covers only a small subset of the larger domain of possible transgressions or failures experienced by people in a given age group. In particular, we intentionally focused on broadly applicable situations and behaviors likely to be encountered by most respondents at some point in their day-to-day life. Our aim was to construct familiar situations that people could easily relate to, so that they could readily imagine themselves in the situations and thereby more accurately report their likely reactions. In fact, the TOSCA and TOSCA-C scenarios and responses were "subject-generated" as opposed to "experimenter-generated." In selecting the scenarios, we drew on narrative accounts of personal shame, guilt, and pride experiences provided by a sample of several hundred college students, noncollege adults, and children. Likewise, the responses to the scenarios were drawn from a much larger pool of affective, cognitive, and behavioral responses provided by a second sample of noncollege adults and children. In selecting scenarios and responses, we purposely favored those that were cited by multiple respondents. One of the advantages of this approach is that we ended up with quite "ecologically valid" measures that are broadly applicable to people in a given age group. But what is missing are less common, more idiosyncratic events (e.g., missing an important medication, behaving insensitively with a mentally ill family member) and more serious transgressions (e.g., hitting a child with a car, losing the family fortune in an ill-advised business deal) that are irrelevant to most respondents but that may dominate a specific person's emotional life at a particular time. Stated another way, our measures assess generalized tendencies to experience shame and guilt across a broad range of everyday situations. They are less apt to capture intense but more circumscribed shame and guilt experiences focused in a specific domain (e.g., failures at dieting, marital infidelity, a vulnerable or stigmatized family member).

A third potential concern has to do with the degree to which scenario-based measures may, in part, *confound shame-proneness and guilt-proneness with moral standards*. As discussed earlier, from a conceptual standpoint, there is good reason to view these as distinct constructs. Shame-proneness and guilt-proneness are affective dispositions, whereas moral standards represent a set of beliefs guiding one's evaluation of behaviors. Citing correlations with their Moral Standards Scale, Kugler and Jones (1992) have suggested that measures referencing specific situations or behaviors are more likely to tap values and standards than the emotion of guilt itself. In Kugler and Jones's view, adjective checklist measures and the guilt scales from their Guilt Inventory more directly tap the "affective experience" of guilt precisely because they omit references to specific situations (e.g., specific moral decisions or dilemmas).

No question, there is some merit to this concern. It is hard to imagine someone enthusiastically endorsing a guilt response to a particular scenario (indicating that he or she would be very likely to feel guilt in that situation) without viewing the eliciting behavior as a violation of his or her standards of conduct. So some degree of moral judgment would seem to be indirectly involved. Although the content of our scenario-based shame and guilt items remains focused on phenomenological descriptions of shame and guilt experiences—not on values, attitudes, and beliefs, as in the Mosher Forced-Choice Guilt Inventory, for example—some moral judgment would typically be a prerequisite for an experience of guilt or shame.

This is a situation where unfortunately researchers cannot have their cake and eat it too. In assessing shame-proneness and guilt-proneness, we are essentially faced with a trade-off. We can either attempt to assess these emotion dispositions by focusing on a checklist of "pure" affective descriptors without reference to specific situations that may muddy the waters with moral judgments. But without these specific situations, the distinction between shame and guilt is more likely to be lost because there is no longer the opportunity to assess guilt about a specific behavior distinct from shame about the self. In our view, scenario-based measures provide a more conceptually sound method for assessing guilt responses, distinct from shame responses, precisely because of their focus on specific situations and behaviors. But, on the down side, the inclusion of specific behaviors invites unwanted variance associated with moral beliefs and standards. In our scenario-based measures, we have tried to minimize a confound with moral standards by (1) focusing on phenomenological descriptions of shame and guilt experiences, rather than cognitive evaluations of whether a particular behavior is "right" or "wrong," and (2) avoiding clearly controversial behaviors (e.g., abortion, premarital sex, eating red meat) on which there is less likely to be moral evaluation consensus. So, in effect, we have attempted to restrict moral judgment variance by selecting situations generally regarded as morally problematic.

Kugler and Jones's (1992) findings suggest that we have been reasonably successful in this regard. Their measure of Moral Standards showed fairly low correlations with the TOSCA Shame and Guilt scales

(.25 and .27, respectively), lower than with the Mosher Guilt scales (.33 to .51), but not as negligible as with the PFQ Shame and Guilt scales (.04 and .14, respectively).

A fourth potential limitation of our scenario-based measures is the degree to which they may fail to tap more "maladaptive" forms of guilt. In Chapter 7, we discuss the issue of adaptive versus maladaptive guilt in greater detail; but to summarize briefly, theories vary widely in their portrayal of guilt as an adaptive versus maladaptive emotion. On the one hand, a long clinical tradition has stressed the pathogenic nature of guilt, emphasizing guilt's role in the formation of many different types of psychological symptoms (e.g., Freud, 1896/1953a, 1924/1961c; Harder, 1995; Harder & Lewis, 1987; Zahn-Waxler & Robinson, 1995). On the other hand, developmental and social psychologists (e.g., Baumeister, Stillwell, & Heatherton, 1994, 1995; Barrett, 1995; Eisenberg, 1986; Hoffman, 1982; Tangney, 1990, 1995a, 1995b, 1995c; Tangney et al., 1995) have stressed the adaptive functions of guilt for moral behavior and social adjustment, particularly in recent years. Baumeister et al. (1994), for example, have presented an elegant theoretical analysis of the relationship-enhancing functions of guilt, drawing on current theory and empirical research.

In Chapters 5, 6, and 7, we present results from studies employing scenario-based measures (e.g., the SCAAI and TOSCA) that generally highlight the positive potential of guilt. Proneness to "shame-free" guilt (i.e., guilt with shame partialed out) is generally unrelated to psychological symptoms but positively correlated with such adaptive dimensions as a capacity for interpersonal empathy, constructive anger management strategies, and benevolent interpersonal perceptions (Petersen et al., 1995; Tangney, 1991, 1994, 1995a, 1995b, 1995c; Tangney, Wagner, & Gramzow, 1992; Tangney, Wagner, et al., 1996). In contrast, studies employing adjective checklist measures generally find little difference in the emotional and social adjustment correlates of shame-proneness and guilt-proneness (Harder & Lewis, 1987; Harder, 1995; Hoblitzelle, 1987).

The scenario-based findings, which underscore guilt's positive potential, make a great deal of sense once one makes the critical distinction between shame and guilt (guilt as a sense of remorse over a specific behavior rather than shame as a global condemnation of the self). The distinction between self and behavior, inherent in guilt, helps people protect the self from unwarranted global devaluation. Perhaps more important, because of this focus on a specific behavior, the path toward constructive change, reparation, and resolution is much clearer. It is much easier to change a bad behavior than to change a bad self.

Nonetheless, the clinical literature suggests that there may be a darker side to guilt as well. And this is an issue that guilt researchers (e.g., Jane Bybee, Sue Crowley, Tamara J. Ferguson, David W. Harder, and our research lab) have begun to take a close look at (e.g., Bybee & Tangney, 1996). Elsewhere, we have suggested that guilt is especially likely to "take a turn for the worse" when it becomes fused with shame (Tangney et al., 1995). From this perspective, it is the shame component of a shame–guilt sequence that sets the stage for psychological symptoms. In Chapter 7, we speculate about additional factors that may render some forms of "shame-free" guilt maladaptive, drawing on recent work by Ferguson, Bybee, Zahn-Waxler, and others.

In our view, this is still an area with many unanswered questions and more empirical work is needed. It is worth noting, however, that our initial efforts to develop a "Maladaptive Guilt" scale for the TOSCA (TOSCA-2; Tangney, Ferguson, Wagner, Crowley, & Gramzow, 1996) argue against a maladaptive guilt distinct from shame.

Several years ago, we created the TOSCA-2, augmenting the TOSCA with a new subscale aimed at tapping a chronic, ruminative, unresolved type of guilt (Tangney, Ferguson, et al., 1996). The Maladaptive Guilt scale includes such responses as "You would walk around for days kicking yourself, thinking of all the mistakes you'd made" and "You would berate yourself over and over for it and vow to *never* do it again." We included the TOSCA-2 in a larger investigation of the psychological and social correlates of moral emotions. A primary interest was to see whether we could tap a Maladaptive Guilt, distinct from Shame.

Results were not encouraging. First, in this study of 381 undergraduates, the correlation between proneness to Maladaptive Guilt and Shame-proneness was $r = .74$. That is about the highest correlation one could expect, given that neither measure is perfectly reliable. This suggests that the two scales are assessing identical constructs. More important, there were no discernable differences in the correlates of Shame and Maladaptive Guilt across a broad range of domains (anxiety, depression, anger and aggression, constructive anger management strategies, self-control, perfectionism, self-esteem, attachment, ego identity, ego strength, fear of negative evaluation, dissociation, embarrassment), other than the fact that the magnitude of effects tended to be stronger for shame.

The TOSCA Measures

Copies of our scenario-based measures—the TOSCA-3, the most recent adult version of our measure (Tangney, Dearing, Wagner, & Gramzow, 2000); the TOSCA-A for adolescents (Tangney, Wagner, Gavlas, & Gramzow, 1991a); and the TOSCA-C for children (Tangney et al., 1990)—appear in Appendix B, along with scoring, reliability, and normative information. Interested readers can also obtain from the first author the original TOSCA (Tangney et al., 1989) and the TOSCA-2 for adults (Tangney, Ferguson, et al., 1996), which includes an experimental "Maladaptive Guilt" scale. In creating the TOSCA-2, we also added two new scenarios and deleted the "dieting" scenario, owing to concerns about gender bias. The most recent version of our measure, the TOSCA-3 (Tangney et al., 2000), eliminates the Maladaptive Guilt items because, as described above, analyses of the Maladaptive Guilt scale have been disappointing. In addition, the TOSCA-3 includes the option of a short version, which drops positive scenarios (and therefore eliminates the Pride scales). In a recent study, short versions of the TOSCA-3 shame and guilt scales correlated .94 and .93 with their corresponding full-length versions, thus supporting the utility of the abbreviated form. Finally, Appendix B includes a version of the TOSCA modified for use with "socially deviant" populations, especially incarcerated individuals (TOSCA-SD; Hanson & Tangney, 1995).

Many of these measures—especially the original TOSCA—have been translated into other languages and are being used in studies of other cultures. The TOSCA, for example, has been translated into Hebrew, Italian, French, German, Hungarian, and Swedish.

STATE MEASURES: FEELINGS OF SHAME AND GUILT IN THE MOMENT

Thus far, we have been focusing on dispositional measures of shame and guilt, assessing individual differences in the tendency to experience one or both of these emotions across a range of situations. Far less work has been done to develop measures of state shame and guilt, but some options are available for researchers interested in studying these emotions "in the moment."

The most widely used measure of state shame and guilt comes from Izard's Differential Emotions Scale (DES; Izard, 1977). Various forms of the DES exist, some relying on single word descriptors of key emotions (e.g., guilt, shyness, sadness) and others drawing on clusters of closely related emotion words to describe each key emotion (e.g., for guilt: repentant, guilty, blameworthy), each rated on a 5-point scale in reference to the respondent's current feeling state. One potential problem with the DES is that shame and embarrassment are merged into a common cluster. Tangney, Miller, et al. (1996) presented evidence that, if anything, shame and embarrassment are even more distinct emotions than shame and guilt. For this reason, researchers may prefer Mosher and White's (1981) modified DES, which presents separate embarrassment and shyness clusters.

The DES measures share some of the same problems with the adjective checklist-type measures described above. Although high in face validity, this approach relies very heavily on respondents' ability to distinguish between the terms "shame" and "guilt." We have made some attempt to circumvent this problem with our State Shame and Guilt Scale (SSGS; Marschall, Sanftner, & Tangney, 1994). The SSGS is composed of brief phenomenological descriptions of shame (5 items, e.g., "I feel humiliated, disgraced," "I want to sink into the floor and disappear") and guilt (5 items, e.g., "I feel remorse, regret," "I cannot stop thinking about something bad I have done") experiences, each rated on a 5-point scale. Nonetheless, without explicitly referring to a specific behavior, there remain some questions about the degree to which this approach can truly tap H. B. Lewis's (1971) shame-about-self versus guilt-about-behavior distinction.

Using a somewhat different approach, Kugler and Jones (1992) have developed a State Guilt Scale as part of their Guilt Inventory. The State Guilt Scale is composed of 10 items such as "I have recently done something that I deeply regret." Like many dispositional measures that do not explicitly attempt to assess and distinguish between shame and guilt, some of the items seem likely to tap shame experiences (e.g., "Lately, it hasn't been easy being me" and "Lately, I have felt good about myself and what I have done") as well as guilt experiences.

More recently, Turner (1998) developed the Experiential Shame Scale (ESS), an inventive measure of state shame explicitly intended to circumvent the inevitable defensive biases inherent in experiencing shame. Recognizing that people are often unable or reluctant to directly acknowledge feelings of shame, Turner (1998) attempted to develop a more "opaque" measure of state shame, purposely reducing the "face validity" of her measure. The ESS is composed of 10 bipolar items tap-ping physical (e.g., "Physically, I feel '1' pale to '7' flushed"), emotional (e.g., "Emotionally, I feel '1' content to '7' distressed"), and social/interpersonal (e.g., "Socially, I feel like '1' hiding to '7' being sociable"—reversed) dimensions of the shame experience. Turner (1998) has presented some promising initial data supporting the reliability and va-lidity of the ESS.

In addition, developmental psychologists have devised methods for assessing behavioral signs of shame and guilt in very young children who have not yet attained the verbal skills necessary to directly report these emotion experiences. Although shame and guilt do not appear to have readily definable facial expressions (Izard, 1977), Barrett, Zahn-Waxler, and Cole (1993) focus on avoiding versus amending behavior as presumed behavioral markers of shame and guilt, respectively. In their "Clown Doll Paradigm," children are given a clown doll, identified as the experimenter's favorite toy, which is rigged to fall apart as the child plays with it. Subsequent behavior is coded as shame-relevant (hiding, avoiding, etc.) or guilt-relevant (attempting to fix, apologizing, etc.). Several other "observational" measures of shame have been devel-oped. To assess young children's feelings of shame and pride, M. Lewis, Alessandri, and Sullivan (1992) focus on facial and postural indicators of these emotions in response to *in vivo* events. Retzinger (1987) has described both verbal and nonverbal markers of adults' experience of shame–rage, and Keltner (1995) has delineated postural markers of shame among adults. And Covert (2000) has developed a comprehen-sive behavioral observation coding system, drawing on previous work by M. Lewis et al. (1992), Retzinger (1987), and Keltner (1995).

Finally, there have been several attempts to develop schemes for coding shame and guilt experiences in narrative accounts and running text. H. B. Lewis (1971), for example, employed Gottschalk and Gleser's (1969) coding system, scoring references to adverse criticism, abuse, moral condemnation, and so forth, as guilt markers, and references to ridicule, inadequacy, shame, embarrassment, humiliation, and so forth, as shame markers. This is an appealing approach because of its poten-tially broad applicability to many types of data: autobiographical narra-tive accounts of real life experiences, transcripts of interpersonal ex-changes, therapy sessions, etc. Unfortunately, evidence for the reliability and validity of such coding schemes has been disappointing (Binder, 1970; Crouppen, 1976; R. L. Smith, 1972), and emotions researchers have largely abandoned these attempts to assess shame and guilt in running text as a result. In our view, more promising future work in this direction seems unlikely using spontaneous, unqueried narrative material, if only because in our experience and in that of other researchers (R. F. Baumeister, personal communication, November 16, 1996; Barrett, Ferguson, Smith, & Bertuzzi, 2000; Ferguson et al., 2000) people rarely articulate shame experiences spontaneously, without pointed inquiry from an interviewer.

SUMMARY AND CONCLUSIONS

In this chapter, we have surveyed the range of measures that have been developed for assessing shame and guilt—both at the dispositional level and at the state or situational level. In doing so, we have tried to summarize some of the key conceptual and methodological issues that face researchers interested assessing these emotions. Table 3.3 summarizes the pros and cons of the most widely used approaches for measuring these moral emotions.

In evaluating the relative strengths and weaknesses of various shame and guilt measures, we considered two issues: First, what *definitions* of shame and guilt underlie a given measure? Empirical research has repeatedly shown that shame and guilt are distinct emotions with very different relationships to many aspects of psychological adjustment and social behavior. For example, it is not unusual to find that the correlations of shame-proneness and guilt-proneness with other constructs differ not just in magnitude but also in *direction*. So when researchers use nonspecific measures of shame/guilt, they may obtain negligible correlations and erroneously interpret shame and guilt as irrelevant, when in fact two important opposing relationships have essentially canceled one another out. Second, given a researcher's definition of shame and guilt, how well does the measure *operationalize* these emotion constructs? Here, we emphasize the importance of both the form and the content of the measure. In our view, the structure of scenario-based measures is most conceptually consistent with current notions of guilt. Guilt is an emotion that stems from a negative evaluation of specific behaviors. So scenario-based methods, describing specific events, seem uniquely well suited for assessing guilt. Unlike global adjective-rating scales that are devoid of specific contexts and behaviors (and thus more

TABLE 3.3. Pros and Cons of Various Approaches to Measuring Shame and Guilt

Shame- versus guilt-inducing situations

Assesses reactions to "shame-inducing" versus "guilt-inducing" situations. Ratings for "shame-inducing" versus "guilt-inducing" situations are aggregated to create indices of shame-proneness and guilt-proneness, respectively.

- *Limitations*: Assumes that shame and guilt are distinguished by differences in the content of eliciting situations. Much research challenges this notion; thus researchers would be well advised to carefully examine the assumptions underlying such measures before selecting this type of assessment.

Global adjective checklists

Checklists of shame- and guilt-related adjectives. Respondents rate how well each adjective describes the self or how frequently they experience such feelings.

- *Advantages*: High face validity; easy to administer.
- *Limitations*: May require very advanced verbal skills; respondents must be able to distinguish between the terms "shame" and "guilt" in the abstract; poses respondents with a shame-like task in the absence of any specific situational context, so it is difficult to assess guilt about specific behaviors separate from the global self.

Scenario-based measures

Respondents are presented with a series of specific common situations, followed by brief phenomenological descriptions of shame and guilt in the specific context.

- *Advantages*: Structure of the measure is more conceptually consistent with current notions of guilt; does not rely on the terms "shame" and "guilt" that may confuse laypersons; less likely to arouse defensiveness.
- *Limitations*: Relatively low internal consistency; constraints on the range of shame- and guilt-inducing situations; potential confound with moral standards.

representative of shame), scenario-based measures assess tendencies to experience guilt about specific behaviors, distinct from shame about the self. For these and other reasons, we advocate the use of scenario-based measures for assessing individual differences in proneness to shame and guilt.

Since the publication of Helen Block Lewis's (1971) *Shame and Guilt in Neurosis*, considerable progress has been made in constructing theoretically meaningful, psychometrically sound measures of shame and guilt—and the body of systematic empirical research on these important emotions has grown accordingly. Looking to the future, however, we can anticipate the development of even more sophisticated assessment strategies as our conceptions of these emotions continue to evolve.

NOTES

1. Discriminant validity refers to the degree to which a measure validly assesses a construct distinct from other different but related constructs. For example, the developer of a test of creativity would want to show that the new test does not simply measure verbal ability.
2. Consider the internal consistency of adjective checklist measures: Harder and Zalma (1990) reported Cronbach's alphas of .78 for the PFQ-2 Shame scale and .72 for the PFQ-2 Guilt scale. Hoblitzelle (1987) reported alphas of .86 for the Shame scale of the Adapted Shame–Guilt Scale (ASGS) and .88 for the ASGS Guilt scale. (The ASGS is a shorter form of the RSGS.) Alphas for the scenario-based TOSCA Shame and Guilt scales tend to be somewhat more modest. For example, in a recent cross-sectional developmental study (Tangney, Wagner, et al., 1996), alphas for the Shame and Guilt scales, respectively, were .74 and .61 for adults (TOSCA), .74 and .69 for college students (TOSCA), .77 and .81 for adolescents (TOSCA-A), and .78 and .83 for children (TOSCA-C).

Chapter 4

OUR "INTRAPERSONAL" RELATIONSHIP
The Self in Shame and Guilt

When we think about relationships, we generally think of our associations and connections with other people. But one of the most important—and certainly most intimate—relationships we have is with our *self*. Each time you look in the mirror, you're faced with your closest ally and, potentially, your greatest enemy. Some people approach themselves with warmth, nurturance, and acceptance. For others, the relationship with the self is fraught with ambivalence, antagonism, and mistrust. Most of us fall somewhere in the middle.

Although the notion of a relationship with oneself may seem a bit odd at first glance, our relationship with our *self* has many of the same characteristics as our relationships with *others*. We have feelings about the self—feelings that fluctuate depending on our recent and past actions. We hold internal dialogues with the self. With time, effort, and experience, we come to know ourselves better.

By their very nature, shame and guilt are fundamentally tied to our perceptions of self. In this chapter, we examine the implications of shame and guilt for our inner experience of the self. We have chosen to focus on this aspect of shame and guilt early in the book because we believe that how shame and guilt affect self-esteem and related self functions can have a substantial impact on the dynamics of interpersonal relationships.

MAKING SENSE OF NEGATIVE EVENTS:
ATTRIBUTING CAUSE, ATTRIBUTING BLAME

In the course of daily life, bad things inevitably happen. Misfortunes befall us and those close to us. Things break. Things get lost. We make mistakes. We fail at important tasks. People become disappointed or annoyed with us. Important relationships dissolve. Pets and plants expire. According to attribution theory, human beings are naturally drawn to search for explanations of these noteworthy events (B. Weiner, 1986). In order to understand these events, we look to many sources: other people, aspects of the environment or situation, divine intervention, fate, dumb luck, and—importantly—ourselves. Assessing the situation, we may blame our spouse for the lost keys. We may blame poor weather for the withering plants. We may blame fate for a broken romance. But when we blame ourselves, we're most apt to feel shame and guilt. Shame and guilt are emotions of self-blame. They are inextricably linked to internal attributions for negative events (events that are judged to be negative based on our own or others' standards).

In fact, the distinction between shame and guilt can be partly captured by contrasting the types of attributions involved in these experiences. Abramson, Seligman, and Teasdale (1978) have identified three dimensions of causal attributions that are particularly useful in this regard: locus (internal vs. external), globality (global vs. specific), and stability (stable vs. unstable). Shame and guilt each involve internal attributions but are likely to vary along the dimensions of globality and stability. To the extent that guilt involves a focus on some specific behavior, the guilt experience is likely to involve internal, specific, and fairly unstable attributions. For example, a young woman may feel guilt for cheating on her boyfriend. Focusing on that *specific* indiscretion, she feels a sense of tension, remorse and regret over what she has *done*. She knows she's responsible; *she* made the ill-advised decision to stray (an internal attribution). But she recognizes that the causes of this transgression are fairly specific; she's not generally a promiscuous or disloyal person (specific attributions to causes that affect only a narrow range of events). Moreover, the factors that led to her infidelity are unique to the current space and time; she sees the causes as variable (unstable attributions).

In contrast, shame involves a focus on the global self, which is presumably relatively enduring. Thus, the shame experience is likely to involve internal, stable, and global attributions. A young man in similar circumstances (cheating on his girlfriend) may feel an acute sense of shame—feeling disgraceful and small, wanting to hide, even disappear. Focusing on *himself*, he knows he is responsible (an internal attribution). Moreover, he views the causes of this transgression as likely to affect many aspects of his life, as characteristic of the type of person he is—disloyal, untrustworthy, immoral, even reprehensible! In short, he makes attributions to quite fundamental features of himself that have much broader implications beyond the specific transgression at hand (global attributions). Finally, he views these factors as persisting across time (stable attributions); he'll be facing the same character flaws tomorrow, and the next day, and the next.

Early in our research on shame and guilt, we examined the links between attributional style and shame-prone and guilt-prone styles (Tangney et al., 1992). In two studies, several hundred undergraduates completed the Attributional Style Questionnaire (ASQ; Seligman, Abramson, Semmel, & von Baeyer, 1979) and our SCAAI measure (the precursor to the TOSCA) assessing individual differences in proneness to shame and proneness to guilt. Students in the second study also completed the TOSCA. The results from both studies clearly showed that shame-proneness is associated with a depressogenic attributional style. People who indicated that they were likely to experience shame across the range of situations described in the SCAAI (and TOSCA) also made many internal, stable, and global attributions for the entirely different set of negative situations described in the ASQ. For example, people who said on the TOSCA that, when criticized for a mistake at work, they would be very likely to "feel like they wanted to hide" (a shame response) were also inclined on the ASQ to attribute a friend's hostility to stable, global aspects of themselves.

It is worth noting, however, that shame-proneness is not the same thing as a depressogenic attributional style. The magnitude of the correlations indicates that these are related but distinct constructs. Moreover, as we discuss in greater detail in Chapter 7, proneness to shame is substantially associated with depressive symptoms *above and beyond* that accounted for by attributional style. Feelings of shame entail a complex array of cognitive, affective, and motivational features (see the discussion of phenomenological studies of shame in Chapter 2). The cluster of depressogenic attributions is just one component of this multifaceted emotional experience. Furthermore, it is possible to make internal, stable, and global attributions for a negative event without an ensuing shame experience. For example, an unemployed middle-aged man who strikes out on yet another job interview might make internal, stable, and global attributions for the fact that he wasn't hired. He may believe that his rejection was due to his poor interviewing skills (an internal attribution), which have always been poor and which are unlikely to change (a stable attribution), and which are pretty general weaknesses that adversely affect his chances for many different jobs (a global attribution). Recognizing all this, he *might* feel shame over his inadequate interviewing skills. But he might instead simply feel a sense of deep disappointment and hopelessness, recognizing that he has strong technical skills, feeling frustrated that his interpersonal awkwardness overshadows his résumé at the critical juncture of a job interview. Internal, stable, and global attributions for negative events set the stage for a shame experience. But they are not invariably linked.

The link between feelings of guilt and internal, unstable, and specific attributions appears more tenuous. In our studies of undergraduates (Tangney, Wagner, & Gramzow, 1992), the attributional style correlates of guilt-proneness did not reflect the expected pattern of results. Proneness to "shame-free" guilt (as assessed by our SCAAI and TOSCA measures) was essentially uncorrelated with internal, unstable, and specific attributions for negative events on the ASQ. Our guess is that these null results are due to at least two factors: First, it seems to us that (compared to ISG—internal, stable, and global—attributions) internal, unstable, and specific attributions for negative events can result in an even broader range of reactions, with guilt being only one such response. In acknowledging one's role in a negative event but conceptualizing it as fairly transient and specific to the particular situation, a person *may* experience guilt (e.g., he or she may earnestly accept responsibility and experience the tension, regret, and remorse over the "bad thing that was done"). But because of the specific and unstable nature of the cause, the person might very well instead downplay the importance of his or her role (e.g., "Well, I did it, but it was only one time and it only caused a problem in this one area"). As a result, there may be little negative affect of any kind. Second, a good proportion of the situations presented in the ASQ don't really lend themselves to feelings of guilt because they describe outcomes, not specific behaviors about which one might feel guilty. For example, a respondent might feel shame upon being rejected for a job owing to the ensuing state of unemployment. But without a more detailed account of the behaviors leading up to the job rejection, the respondent would really have to "fill in the blanks" to imagine a guilt reaction. Thus, the absence of a link

between guilt-proneness and an internal, unstable, and specific attributional style may be due in part to the nature of the items on the ASQ. A
similar measure with richer descriptions of events, including specific
behaviors, would probably be more sensitive in detecting the hypothesized relationship between guilt experiences and internal, unstable, and
specific attributions.

Finally, it is worth mentioning that the cognitive attributional components of shame and guilt also parallel Janoff-Bulman's (1979) distinction between characterological versus behavioral self-blame. Theoretically, shameful feelings (about the self) are most closely linked to
characterological self-blame; guilty feelings (about specific behaviors)
are most closely linked to behavioral self-blame. It is interesting to note
that one of Janoff-Bulman's key propositions concerns the relative utility of behavioral versus characterological self-blame. From Janoff-
Bulman's perspective, behavioral self-blame represents a more adaptive
response to traumatic events (e.g., Janoff-Bulman focused on patterns of
blame among rape victims) because one can change specific behaviors
in future circumstances (say, avoiding poorly lit parking garages). Thus,
behavioral self-blame can lead to a greater sense of control over subsequent events. Empirical research on the implications of behavioral versus characterological self-blame has been rather mixed. But these ideas
parallel a theme presented throughout the remainder of this book—
namely, that on balance feelings of guilt are more adaptive than feelings
of shame as we are confronted with our inevitable failures and transgressions.

SHAME AND SELF-ESTEEM

What Is the Difference between Shame and
Low Self-Esteem?

Feelings of shame involve an affective reaction to a global negative
evaluation of the self. But how does shame differ from low self-esteem?
Although feelings of shame likely play an important role in problems of
self-esteem, these are nonetheless distinct constructs. Global self-
esteem is a stable trait involving one's general evaluation of the self,
largely independent of specific situations. Theoretical definitions vary
in their emphasis on affective and cognitive components; some approaches also consider self-esteem in fairly general domains (e.g.,
physical appearance, academics). But self-esteem is essentially a self-

evaluative construct representing how a person appraises him- or herself, in general, across situations over time.

Shame, on the other hand, is an emotion—an affective state. The *feeling* of shame involves a negative evaluation of the global self, but one that is in response to a specific failure or transgression, not necessarily reflective of one's general level of self-esteem. The corresponding trait or disposition is *shame-proneness*, a tendency to experience the emotion shame (as opposed to, say, guilt) in response to specific negative events.

And, in fact, the correlation between shame-proneness and self-esteem is fairly modest. The relationship between shame-proneness and self-esteem is consistently negative. But the magnitude of the relationship is not huge—on average $r = -.42$ for adults. Thus, these constructs are related but distinct. Although people who are inclined to feel shame in response to specific negative events are also, on balance, somewhat likely to have low self-esteem, this is not a one-to-one relationship. The modest correlation allows for various individual combinations of shame/self-esteem attributes. (See Appendix A, Table A.2, for more detailed results on the relationship of self-esteem to shame-proneness and guilt-proneness from multiple studies of children, adolescents, and adults.)

For example, Figure 4.1 illustrates four possible scenarios. Figure 4.1a shows the hypothetical profile of Bill—a low self-esteem, shame-prone individual. In general, Bill doesn't think particularly well of himself. On any given day, he is likely to compare himself unfavorably to others. But, in addition, Bill is prone to frequent episodes of shame. When he makes a mistake, forgets an appointment, or hurts his son's feelings, Bill very often feels that painful wash of shame, that sense of shrinking and being small, wanting to disappear. In effect, these shame experiences are affectively loaded, sudden but transient drops in self-esteem.[1]

Consider, in contrast, Carmen—a high self-esteem, shame-prone individual (Figure 4.1b). In general, Carmen has a positive view of herself. She sees herself as a competent, likable, and worthy person. But like Bill, Carmen is prone to experience shame when she fails or transgresses. She's inclined to rather dramatic but transient drops in self-regard that come with the acute pain of shame. Fortunately, life moves on. As Carmen recovers from such shame episodes, so does her self-regard.

Non-shame-prone people can also be either high or low in self-

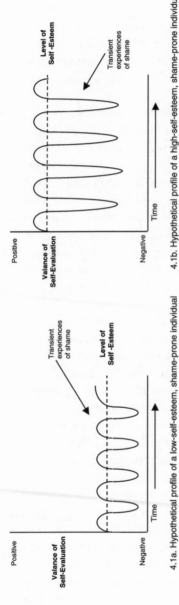

4.1a. Hypothetical profile of a low-self-esteem, shame-prone individual

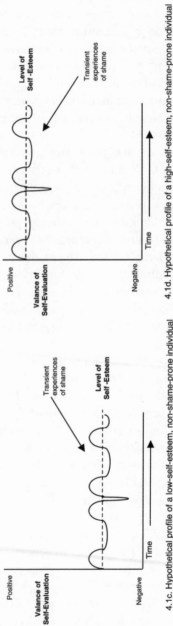

4.1b. Hypothetical profile of a high-self-esteem, shame-prone individual

4.1c. Hypothetical profile of a low-self-esteem, non-shame-prone individual

4.1d. Hypothetical profile of a high-self-esteem, non-shame-prone individual

FIGURE 4.1. Shame and self-esteem.

58

esteem. Figure 4.1c shows the hypothetical profile of Janet—a low self-esteem, non-shame-prone individual. In general, Janet doesn't think particularly well of herself. But shame is not her characteristic reaction to failures and transgressions. Similarly, Tyrone (Figure 4.1d), a high-self-esteem individual, isn't much plagued by the distress of shame.

Bill and Tyrone's profiles fit the majority of people, as indicated by the mean correlation of $r = -.42$ between shame-proneness and self-esteem. But the correlation is not $r = -.80$. There are plenty of high-self-esteem, shame-prone people and low-self-esteem, non-shame-prone people in the world![2]

What Are the Dynamics between Shame and Self-Esteem?

Why do shame-prone people tend to have somewhat lower self-esteem than their non-shame-prone peers? Thus far, research in this area has been exclusively correlational. We have no hard data on the causal nature of the link between shame and self-esteem. But we speculate that the relationship between shame and self-esteem is complex, involving bidirectional influences. Moreover, there are undoubtedly a number of personality characteristics that moderate this link between shame-proneness and level self-esteem.

On the one hand, proneness to the ugly feeling of shame can lead to deficits in self-esteem. That is, frequent and repeated experiences of shame are apt to "chip away" at one's general level of self-regard over the long haul. As we've discussed, in an attempt to find explanations for the inevitable negative events in everyday life, people not infrequently look to the self as a fundamental cause—feeling shame or guilt, or some combination of these emotions in the face of self-blame. The self is a living, reactive, dynamic entity that responds to these cognitive-affective self-references. Blaming the self for significant failures or transgressions poses a threat to our self-image. As we discuss in subsequent chapters, such ego threats may motivate actions ranging from proactive change to defensive avoidance. But, in addition, over time, such ego threats are also likely to have implications for our more general level of self-esteem, particularly if one is prone to respond with feelings of shame about the self rather than feelings of guilt about a specific behavior.

Feelings of shame pose the most serious threat to self-esteem because it is the self, not a specific behavior, that is the focus of negative evaluation. In contrast, the guilt experience represents a less profound challenge to one's enduring self because what's at issue is a specific behavior somewhat apart from the global self. As shown in greater detail in Appendix A (Table A.2), across numerous studies of children, adolescents, and adults, proneness to guilt was generally uncorrelated with self-esteem. In fact, the part correlations indicate that, if anything, proneness to "shame-free guilt" (the unique variance in guilt, independent of shame) is *positively* correlated with self-esteem. Thus, it appears that repeated experiences of shame, but not guilt, are apt to erode one's overall evaluation of the self.

For example, 27-year-old Robert—a participant in one of our undergraduate research studies—related this shame experience:

" . . . when I was reprimanded by a supervisor at work in front of all my coworkers. I incorrectly performed a part of a project I was working on which other people based their work on. Everyone was upset, and I felt totally humiliated in front of everyone. It took me months to regain self-composure, confidence. My work, personality, self-esteem suffered immensely."

At the same time, it seems likely that low self-esteem sets the stage for frequent and repeated experiences of shame. Imagine the experience of Bill, our low self-esteem individual, as he faces yet another of the inevitable blunders of everyday life. Bill just realized that he inadvertently made his coworker, John, look bad in a memo to their boss. Bill generally thinks rather poorly of himself. In his heart of hearts, he sees himself as pretty much of a bumbling, thoughtless, less-than-competent oaf. In his automatic search for the meaning of his error at work, what do you suppose stands out as the most salient cause? Is it his characteristic, enduring, bumbling, and inadequate self? Or is it a more specific transient set of factors leading to this specific misguided behavior? Our guess is that low self-esteem individuals are drawn to blame their "bad self" when faced with negative events.

So far, we have been suggesting that feelings of shame engender low self-esteem and, in turn, low self-esteem results in a vulnerability to feelings of shame. Why then are some high-self-esteem people shame-prone? And why are some low-self-esteem people relatively immune to shame experiences? Clearly with an $r = -.42$ correlation between self-esteem and shame-proneness, the relationship isn't absolute. Our guess is that there are at least three sets of factors that influence or moderate the link between shame and self-esteem. Figure 4.2 illustrates the direct bidirectional effects between shame and self-esteem, as well as the various psychological and social factors that may enhance or attenuate this link. Paths *a* and *b* represent the direct effects of shame on self-esteem and vice versa, already discussed. Certainly, however, there are other factors that affect people's self-esteem besides their proneness to shame (see path *c*). They may have a variety of assets that contribute directly to their level of self-esteem: a history of academic success, other unusual skills or abilities, respect and approval from significant others, etc. Such positive attributes are especially likely to enhance a person's self-esteem when they represent self-relevant dimensions valued by that individual. On the flip side of the coin, people are often encumbered by perceived deficits of various sorts that can lower their self-regard (e.g., cognitive deficits, physical unattractiveness, poor social skills, membership in an oppressed minority group). Again, such seemingly negative attributes are especially likely to diminish an individual's self-regard when they are in personally valued domains (Tesser, 1999).

On the other side of Figure 4.2, there are numerous factors that shape a person's propensity to experience shame beyond low self-esteem (path *d*). In Chapter 9, we discuss the development of moral

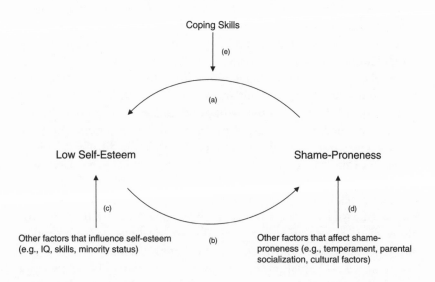

FIGURE 4.2. Factors that may influence the link between shame-proneness and low self-esteem.

affective styles in greater detail. But, in short, we speculate that an individual's tendency to experience shame and/or guilt is influenced by a broad range of factors including early temperament, parental (and other) socialization factors, and cultural environment. One can imagine such effects on a person's proneness to shame independent of self-esteem.

Finally, there is a collection of skills or attributes that may directly affect the degree to which shame-proneness may contribute to low self-esteem (path e's effect on path a). It seems likely that some people are better than others at coping with and recovering from experiences of shame. For example, Carmen, our high-self-esteem, shame-prone person (Figure 4.1b), is inclined to respond to transgressions and failures with acute painful episodes of shame. She may feel for the moment like a worthless and flawed person. But such profound and repeated shame experiences may not adversely affect her more general level of self-regard because she has well-developed skills for recovering from these emotional low points. At present, there is virtually no research on the ways in which people manage their feelings of shame and guilt. But we can speculate that there may be a variety of useful strategies for dispelling feelings of shame—some cognitively oriented, some affectively based, and some socially derived.

Consider two possible cognitive strategies for resolving feelings of shame. Carmen may have learned to counter her shame experiences with "corrective" self-talk, reminding herself that she isn't, after all, a selfish lout of a person just because she declined to help a friend move last weekend. She may deliberately remind herself of all the generous ways she has helped her friends in the past. (In fact, this is the sort of strategy fostered by cognitive-behavioral therapies.) Alternately, she may have learned to "externalize" the blame of shame, rationalizing that her boss's demands for overtime (coupled with her bad back) have prevented her from going to her friend's aid. A more affectively based strategy might involve engaging in a pleasurable and/or pride-inducing activity, reestablishing her connection with more positive domains of self-esteem. And a social strategy might involve "talking through" the failure or transgression and associated shame feelings, seeking support and reassurance from a trusted friend or family member.

Tesser's self-evaluation maintenance (SEM) model (1999; Tesser & Campbell, 1980, 1983) suggests additional tactics for diffusing feelings of shame. According to SEM theory, when making social comparisons, people engage in a variety of psychological maneuvers in order to maintain positive self-regard. When outperformed by another, people may strategically alter the importance they place on the domain of the performance. They may alter their evaluations of others' performance in those domains and their perceptions of the closeness of relationships with others with whom they are compared. In short, some individuals may be more inclined to use "self-evaluation maintenance" tactics than others, strategically altering their perceptions relevant to the context in which they fail or "fall short" in comparison to others.

In the context of shame, the relative effectiveness of such cognitive, affective, and social strategies has yet to be evaluated. But it's a safe bet that there are individual differences not only in proneness to shame but also in people's capacity to resolve feelings of shame when they occur. And this capacity to manage shame episodes, in turn, is likely to moderate the link between proneness to shame and self-esteem.

SELF-AWARENESS, SELF-CONSCIOUSNESS, AND SELF-MONITORING

Shame and guilt are self-conscious emotions. Each centers on negative evaluations of the self or the behavior of the self. In fact, one could argue that shame is the quintessential self-conscious emotion. One feature of shame that stands out in the phenomenological studies summarized in Chapter 2 is the highly self-focused nature of this emotion. At its heart, shame is a self-involved, egocentric experience. The person in the midst of the shame reaction is concerned not so much with the implications for *others* of his or her failure or transgression; he or she is more concerned with the implications of negative events for the *self*.

Social psychologists have developed a fairly extensive literature on self-focused phenomena such as self-awareness, self-consciousness, and self-monitoring. Researchers haven't yet integrated the study of moral emotions with these concepts of self-focused attention, but it seems likely that these inner-directed experiences would be related to people's tendencies to experience shame and guilt.

At any given moment, a person may be more or less self-focused. That is, an individual's attention can be directed inward toward the self or directed outward toward the environment (or someplace in between). The term "self-awareness," coined by Duval and Wicklund (1972), refers to inner-directed attention. Self-awareness is a state—the experience of directing one's attention inward in the moment (see Figure 4.3). "Self-consciousness" refers to the trait, or tendency, to be self-aware. Based on factor analytic results, Fenigstein, Scheier, and Buss (1975) differentiated between public and private self-consciousness: *Public self-consciousness* refers to an individual's tendency to be concerned with the impression that he or she makes on others; a person high on the trait of public self-consciousness is therefore concerned with self-presentation and his or her behavior in social settings. On the other hand, *private self-consciousness* refers to an individual's propensity to be reflective, insightful, and aware of his or her own thoughts and emotions.

Our guess is that when people are in a state of heightened self-awareness, they are a few steps closer to an experience of shame. In fact, research has shown a link between self-focus and tendencies to make attributions about the self. Duval and Wicklund (1973) developed an elegantly simple technique for inducing the state of self-awareness—

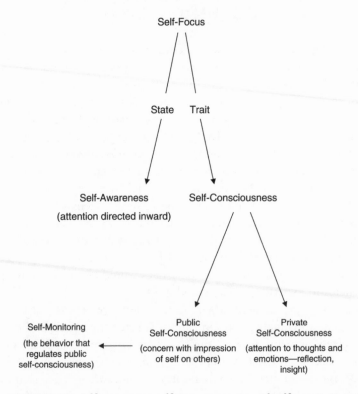

FIGURE 4.3. Self-awareness, self-consciousness, and self-monitoring.

merely confronting research participants with their own image in a mirror. Their results indicate that when the self is the focus of attention, an individual is more likely to attribute causes of both positive and negative events to the self (Duval & Wicklund, 1973). Moreover, this effect of self-focused awareness on self-attributions appears to be most pronounced in the case of negative events (Buss & Scheier, 1976). Taken together, these findings suggest that induced self-awareness may render people more vulnerable to self-blaming feelings of shame. Similarly, research has shown that people high on the trait of self-consciousness—specifically public self-consciousness—are also likely to be shame-prone.[3]

Similar to the idea of public self-consciousness is the concept of self-monitoring. A person's concern with impression management (public self-consciousness) is related to the behavior of self-monitoring. Self-monitoring refers to an individual's attentiveness to interpersonal cues, sensitivity to the dynamics of the situation, and awareness of appropriate social norms (Snyder, 1974; Snyder & Cantor, 1980). Using this information, people who are high in the trait of self-monitoring are better able to adapt their own behavior to a given situation. Similarly, individuals who are high self-monitors tend to place more importance on self-presentation, specifically on how others view them. These individuals are prone to see environmental factors as the cause of their own behavior, and therefore they demonstrate more cross-situational variability in their behavior (Snyder & Swann, 1976).

High self-monitors may be more vulnerable to shame experiences owing to their increased public self-consciousness. Alternately, one might hypothesize that these individuals would be less shame-prone because they would tend to interpret a personal transgression as their reaction to transient situational factors, rather than an inherent fault of their character. In contrast, the behavior of an individual who is low in self-monitoring is more likely to be guided by dispositional characteristics, rather than social cues. These individuals are more committed to their beliefs, standards, and ideals, and less directed by how others view them. Consequently, these individuals are more likely to assume personal responsibility for their own actions. It is possible, then, that when low self-monitors transgress, they tend to view the action as a reflection of themselves, and thus would likely experience shame as a result.

Data from a study of 361 undergraduates supported a modest link between guilt-proneness and self-monitoring. In contrast, the hypothesized negative correlation between shame-proneness and self-monitoring was negligible. Thus, it seems that there is a relationship between feelings of guilt and the tendency to monitor one's behavior, whereas the link between feelings of shame and self-monitoring are less clear. However, these findings are only based on one study, and further research is needed.[4]

BELIEFS ABOUT THE SELF: ENTITY VERSUS INCREMENTAL THEORIES AND SELF–BEHAVIOR CONGRUENCE

In an attempt to understand factors that contribute to individual differences in proneness to shame and guilt, we have also considered people's "beliefs about the self." Although not typically articulated, people develop implicit psychological theories in many domains of human experience. These "theories" then guide each person's interpretations of events, shape his or her affective experiences, and influence interpersonal interactions. People's implicit theories of the self seem especially relevant to the experience of shame and guilt.

Carol S. Dweck and her colleagues at Columbia University (Dweck & Leggett, 1988; Dweck, Hong, & Chiu, 1993) have examined beliefs about the degree to which core traits are fixed versus malleable. Some people view key traits as quite entrenched (entity theorists), whereas others view core characteristics of the self as more flexible and amenable to change (incremental theorists). Dweck and colleagues' research has shown that these beliefs affect behaviors in a number of contexts. Most notably, when faced with failure in achievement settings, entity theorists often "hit a wall," experiencing high degrees of negative affect, feeling helpless, and withdrawing from the task at hand. In contrast, incremental theorists tend to respond to failures with a problem-solving focus, remaining motivated to overcome their initial errors, exerting greater effort, and flexibly experimenting with alternative strategies.

In addition, we've identified a second set of potentially relevant beliefs concerning *self–behavior congruence* (Tangney, Fee, Reinsmith, Bowling, & Yerington, 1997). People vary in the degree to which they believe there is a correspondence between self and behavior. At one extreme, people may subscribe to the notion that "You are what you do" and "A person is best revealed by his or her actions." At the other extreme is the notion that there can be a considerable disjoint between one's self and one's behavior—that people's behavior can be an inaccurate sign of who they really are underneath.

What We Expected

We've conducted some preliminary studies on these "beliefs about the self" (Tangney et al., 1997). Our primary interest centered on the implications of these beliefs for people's moral affective style—specifically their tendencies to experience shame and guilt. We anticipated that people who hold the belief that the self is fixed (as opposed to malleable) as well as the belief that behavior is a strong indicator of character or self (high self–behavior congruence) would be especially vulnerable to feelings of shame (Figure 4.4, quadrant A). Owing to their implicit theories of the self, they would be likely to interpret a single transgression or failure as a sign of a more global failing of the self (self–behavior congruence), a failing of the self that is likely to persist over time (self is fixed). In short, having failed or transgressed, such people may be especially likely to have the shame-filled experience of shrinking and being small, focusing on the belief that they are defective or unworthy.

In contrast, we anticipated that proneness to guilt (about specific behaviors) would be associated with low self–behavior congruence beliefs and perceptions of the self as malleable (Figure 4.4, quadrant D). In the face of failure or transgression, such people may experience the tension, remorse, and regret of guilt over a specific behavior. But they would not be particularly inclined to feel shame about the self.

To evaluate these hypotheses, we constructed brief scales assessing the belief that the self is fixed versus malleable (Self is Fixed, 8 items, a modified version of the self-report measure constructed by Dweck and colleagues) and the belief that self and behavior are congruent versus

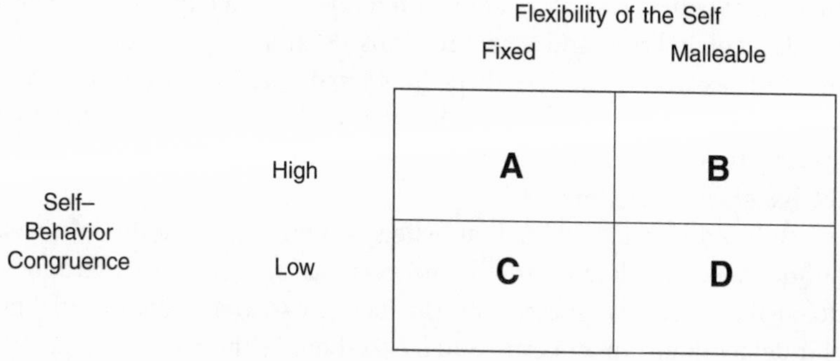

| | | Flexibility of the Self | |
		Fixed	Malleable
Self–Behavior Congruence	High	A	B
	Low	C	D

FIGURE 4.4. Beliefs about the self.

incongruent (Self–Behavior Congruence, 16 items). We considered the possibility that people's beliefs about the nature of their personal self may be different from their beliefs about people's selves in general. Thus, we constructed two versions of each scale—one regarding the *personal self*, and one regarding *others' selves*—yielding four Beliefs About the Self (BAS) subscales. We then asked 175 undergraduates to complete the BAS as well as a number of other measures including our TOSCA scale of proneness to shame and guilt.

What We Found

Our results indicated that the BAS subscales were reliable and that the two sets of beliefs (self is fixed vs. malleable, and self–behavior congruence) were essentially uncorrelated, tapping distinct beliefs about the self. There was a strong correspondence between beliefs about the personal self and beliefs about others' selves. That is, respondents' implicit theories of the self were quite general, pertaining to other people as well as themselves.

Regarding proneness to guilt, our hypotheses were partially borne out. The belief that the self is fixed was negatively correlated with guilt-proneness. That is, people prone to feelings of guilt about specific behaviors (somewhat apart from the self) tended to view the self as relatively flexible and amenable to change. Contrary to expectation, however, there was no relationship between self–behavior congruence beliefs and proneness to guilt. People prone to guilt were no more or less likely to believe that there can be a disjoint between who you are and what you do.

Regarding proneness to shame, we were really off the mark! Neither set of beliefs was correlated with tendencies to experience shame in the face of failures and transgressions. Shame-prone people were no more or less likely to view the self as fixed, and they were no more or less likely to believe "You are what you do." Such cognitive beliefs are apparently insufficient by themselves to render people vulnerable to affective shame reactions.

It is worth mentioning that beliefs about the malleability of the self, although uncorrelated with shame, *were* associated with two types of defensive reactions assessed by the TOSCA—externalization of blame and detachment/unconcern. When asked about their likely response to everyday failures and transgressions, people who believe the self is fixed were inclined to (1) blame other people for these events and/or

(2) adopt a detached, unconcerned attitude (e.g., "It wasn't a big deal, anyway"). As discussed in greater detail in Chapter 6, defensive externalization of blame has been linked to experiences of shame, across numerous studies.

Unanticipated results, like those from our Beliefs About the Self study, are an exciting part of the research process. They remind us that it's important to actually gather data! And they lead us to take a second look at our assumptions and conceptualizations. For example, we are now rethinking the implications of beliefs about self–behavior congruence, based on other results from this preliminary study. Contrary to our expectations, a belief in high self–behavior congruence was moderately *positively* associated with indices of social and psychological adjustment. Apparently, the belief that "You are what you do" doesn't leave people with a sense of helplessness and hopelessness over the dire implications of their failures and transgressions. Rather, it appears to be adaptive to perceive continuity between one's self and one's behavior.

In retrospect, we speculate that perceptions of *low* self–behavior congruence may signify some weakness in the integrity of the self. It would be useful in future research to examine the relationship of these beliefs to indices of ego strength, identity formation, and proneness to dissociative experiences, as well as the degree to which these beliefs moderate the link between shame and self-esteem.

SHAME, GUILT, AND SELF-DISCREPANCIES

We recently examined another set of self-related factors—self-discrepancies—hypothesized to be relevant to individual differences in proneness to shame and guilt (Tangney, Niedenthal, Covert, & Barlow, 1998). Shame and guilt are moral emotions that arise from discrepancies between standards (morally or socially prescribed) and aspects of our behavior or ourselves. Numerous psychological theories (e.g., Epstein, 1980; Heider, 1958; Osgood & Tannenbaum, 1955) have suggested that people typically feel distress when they experience dissonance, imbalance, incongruity, or self-inconsistency. But E. T. Higgins's (1987) self-discrepancy theory is unique in attempting to identify specific types of incompatible or inconsistent beliefs about the self that relate to specific types of negative emotional responses.

At the heart of self-discrepancy theory are two dimensions of self-representation: *domains of the self* and *standpoints on the self*. According to Higgins (1987), there are three basic domains of the self: (1) the *actual* self—attributes that either a person or a significant other believes that the person actually possesses; (2) the *ideal* self—attributes that a person or significant other would like the person ideally to possess (i.e., representation of hopes, wishes); and (3) the *ought* self—attributes that a person or significant other believes the person should or ought to possess (i.e., representations of duty, responsibility).

The standpoint dimension represents the point of view or source of evaluation of the self. Self-discrepancy theory focuses on two standpoints on the self: (1) one's *own* standpoint, and (2) the standpoint (or point of view) of significant *others*.

When the domains of the self are combined with the standpoints on the self, six basic types of self-state representations result: actual/own, actual/other, ideal/own, ideal/other, ought/own, and ought/other. The first two, the actual self-representations, constitute what is usually referred to as the self-concept. The remaining four combinations represent "self-guides."

Self-discrepancy theory focuses primarily on chronic discrepancies between self-concept and self-guides in predicting distinct discrepancy-induced emotional syndromes (Higgins, 1987). In a nutshell, the theory posits that specific types of self-discrepancies (discrepancies between actual self representations and a particular prescriptive "self-guide") are differentially linked to specific types of emotional distress. Most relevant here, self-discrepancy theory predicts that actual/own versus ideal/other discrepancies should result in a tendency to experience shame whereas actual/own versus ought/own discrepancies should lead to a tendency to experience guilt (Higgins, 1987).

Actual/own versus ideal/other discrepancies are present when an individual's actual attributes (from his or her own standpoint) differs from the ideal state that a significant other wishes or hopes the person to attain. According to Higgins (1987), this type of discrepancy results in a vulnerability to dejection-related emotions marked by an absence of positive outcomes (i.e., not obtaining the goals of significant others). More specifically, people with high actual/own versus ideal/other discrepancies are inclined to perceive their significant others as disappointed in or dissatisfied with them, and so should be disposed to react with shame, embarrassment, and feeling downcast. For example, 18-year-old Joan views herself as intelligent, hard-working, shy, and single (how she "actually" is, from her own perspective—actual/own). She believes her parents would ideally like her to be intelligent, hard-working, outgoing, and married (ideal/other). According to Higgins, shame is likely to result from Joan's recognition of the discrepancy between her actual self and what important others would like her to be (shy vs. outgoing; single vs. married).

Actual/own versus ought/own discrepancies arise when a person's actual attributes (from his or her own standpoint) differ from the state that the person feels he or she should or ought to attain. According to Higgins (1987), this type of discrepancy is associated with agitation-related emotions, especially a vulnerability to feelings of guilt, self-contempt, and agitation. Higgins (1987) also suggested that this discrepancy may be associated with feelings of moral weakness and worthlessness. For example, in Joan's case, her view of herself as intelligent, hard-working, shy, and single (actual/own), differs from her personal belief that she should be fun loving, intelligent enough not to have to work too hard, outgoing, and single (ought/own). According to Higgins, this type of discrepancy (actual/own vs. ought/own) between her actual self and what she thinks she ought to be (fun loving vs. hard-working; outgoing vs. shy) is more likely to result in feelings of guilt.

Although Higgins's (1987) hypotheses are intriguing, a closer look at current perspectives on shame and guilt (see Chapter 2) suggested to us an alternative pattern of results. As discussed by H. B. Lewis (1971), feelings of shame involve fairly global negative evaluations of the self— the sense that "*I* am an inferior, inadequate, unworthy (or bad, immoral, unprincipled) person." Guilt, in contrast, involves more circumscribed negative evaluations of specific behaviors (the sense that "I *did* a bad, immoral, unprincipled *thing*"), without necessarily carrying implications for the entire self. Thus, it follows that *self*-discrepancies of all types (e.g., discrepancies between the perceived actual self and any one of a number of "self-guides") would be associated with a tendency to experience the *self*-condemnation of shame. In fact, it wasn't clear to us why one type of self-discrepancy would be any more relevant than another self-discrepancy to feelings of shame about the self. On the other hand, guilt involves a focus on a specific behavior, not the global self. Thus, feelings of guilt are apt to be less centrally relevant to the self than shame. Accordingly, we expected proneness to guilt to be negligibly related to all types of self-discrepancies.

And this is exactly what we found! We asked 229 undergraduates to complete our TOSCA measure of proneness to shame and guilt, and two versions of Higgins's Selves Questionnaire, assessing the various self-discrepancies (Tangney et al., 1998). Consistent with our predictions, but in contrast to Higgins (1987), there was a significant positive relationship between all types of self-discrepancies and the tendency to experience shame. Guilt-proneness, on the other hand, was essentially unrelated to any of the self-discrepancies.[5]

NARCISSISM

Finally, no chapter on shame and the self would be complete without a consideration of narcissism. In recent years, shame has become a "hot topic" in psychoanalytic circles, and quite a number of psychoanalytically oriented clinicians have discussed the special link between shame and narcissism (Kernberg, 1975; Kohut, 1971; H. B. Lewis, 1971, 1987b; Mollon, 1984; A. P. Morrison, 1983, 1989; Wurmser, 1987). In this area, too, the distinction between shame and guilt is important. Theoretically, shame is more centrally relevant to the narcissistic process than guilt because shame and narcissism share a common focus on self-related issues.

At the heart of the narcissistic disorder is a disorder of the self-system (Kernberg, 1975; Kohut, 1971; A. P. Morrison, 1989) involving problems with the regulation of self-esteem, as well as fundamental defects in the formation of a coherent sense of self. H. B. Lewis (1987b) and Wurmser (1987) have suggested that the tenuous self-system of narcissists renders them especially vulnerable to painful self-focused experiences of shame. Moreover, narcissists typically develop many unrealistic expectations for themselves and others that, in effect, set the stage for experiences of shame. With each failure to achieve ambitions— ambitions that are often grandiose—the narcissistic individual is apt to feel shame. Similarly, with each failure to have highly unrealistic needs and expectations gratified by an idealized other, shame is a likely outcome (A. P. Morrison, 1983; Siomopoulus, 1988). Ironically, H. B. Lewis (1987b) speculated that many features of narcissism (e.g., grandiosity, excessive need for admiration from others) are developed as defenses to ward off the dreaded shame reaction. Unfortunately for the narcissist, these defenses are often unsuccessful.

Although the clinical literature abounds with theoretical discussions of the link between shame and narcissism, researchers have only begun to examine this relationship. In one of the earliest studies on this topic, Harder and Lewis (1987) examined the relationship of shame-proneness and guilt-proneness (as assessed by their Personal Feelings

Questionnaire) to narcissism (as assessed by Raskin & Hall's [1979], Narcissistic Personality Inventory, NPI). Their results indicated that guilt-proneness was unrelated to narcissism and, contrary to theory, shame-proneness was *negatively* correlated with narcissism. This negative relationship between shame and narcissism was surprising, to say the least, especially in light of so much clinical observation and theory to the contrary. One possibility is that the rather dramatic defenses inherent in narcissism are in fact quite effective in short-circuiting shame-like reactions. Highly narcissistic individuals may not frequently experience shame. A second possibility, however, is that these theoretically inconsistent results are an artifact of difficulties in the measurement of both narcissism and shame and guilt. For example, Harder and Lewis (1987) speculated that, in asking participants to provide global self-reports of shame-like reactions (e.g., directly asking subjects to rate the frequency or degree to which they experience shame), the PFQ may invite a defensive denial on the part of some respondents (see Chapter 3 for a more extended discussion of issues in the assessment of shame and guilt). Consistent with this notion, H. B. Lewis (1971) and others have observed that some clients frequently repress or deny shame experiences whereas others may not recognize the shame experience as such. This may be particularly the case for narcissistic individuals.

Gramzow and Tangney (1992) subsequently conducted a study employing an entirely different strategy to assess proneness to shame and guilt—the scenario-based SCAAI and TOSCA measures. In Chapter 3, we discussed several advantages of the scenario-based approach. Most relevant here, the SCAAI and TOSCA measures seem better suited to circumvent defensiveness because respondents are asked to rate phenomenological descriptions of components of shame and guilt experiences *with respect to specific situations*, rather than being asked to bluntly acknowledge global tendencies to experience shame and guilt.

Gramzow and Tangney (1992) also struggled with difficulties in the measurement of narcissism. The NPI was developed to assess narcissistic personality features in a *nonclinical* population (Raskin & Hall, 1979, 1981; Raskin & Terry, 1988). Results from a number of studies support the validity of the NPI. For example, total NPI scores have been associated with dominance and exhibitionism (Emmons, 1984; Raskin & Terry, 1988), low interpersonal empathy (Watson, Grisham, Trotter, & Biderman, 1984), frequent use of first person singular nouns (Raskin & Shaw, 1988), and observers' ratings of narcissism (Raskin & Terry, 1988). Still, there is some question about the degree to which the NPI assesses pathological narcissism as typically understood in the clinical literature. For example, Watson et al. (1984) reported *no* relationship between the NPI and the Narcissistic Personality Disorder Scale (Solomon, 1982) derived from the MMPI. Similarly, Mullins and Kopelman (1988) found little convergence between the NPI and three less widely used measures of pathological narcissism. In addition, total NPI scores have been related to positive aspects of adjustment, such as high self-esteem, a high level of congruence between the self and ideal self, low neuroticism, low anxiety, and low depression (Emmons, 1984; Raskin & Terry, 1988; Raskin & Novacek, 1989; Watson, Taylor, & Morris, 1987). These findings are consistent with the notion that, generally speaking, the NPI taps adaptive as opposed to maladaptive aspects of narcissism.

To address these concerns, several researchers have examined factor scores to differentiate between adaptive and pathological components of narcissism on the NPI. Emmons's (1984) factor analysis appears to be most useful in isolating the maladaptive elements of narcissism. The results of several studies (Emmons, 1984; Watson et al., 1987) indicate that three of the factors (Leadership/Authority, Superiority/Arrogance, and Self-Absorption/Self-Admiration) assess primarily benign aspects of the narcissistic personality, while a fourth factor (Exploitativeness/Entitlement) assesses more pathological narcissistic features. Examining the factor correlates of self-esteem and depression, Watson et al. (1987) found this differentiation most apparent when Exploitativeness was partialed out from the three more adaptive factors, and vice versa.

In their study of undergraduates, Gramzow and Tangney (1992) examined the relationship of shame-proneness and guilt-proneness (as assessed by the SCAAI and TOSCA) to total NPI scores and the four Emmons (1984) factors. Following Watson et al. (1987), we used partial correlations to examine the affective correlates of maladaptive narcissism (Exploitativeness) independent of the apparently more adaptive components of narcissism, and vice versa. The results supported the notion that shame-proneness is positively related to pathological aspects of narcissism but negatively related to healthy narcissistic features. When both the SCAAI and TOSCA were considered, the unique variance in shame was positively correlated with Exploitativeness, independent of the apparently more adaptive components of narcissism. In contrast, Leadership and Self-Absorption residuals were consistently negatively correlated with shame. The relationship of guilt-proneness to aspects of narcissism was less consistent—but, where significant, guilt residuals were correlated with narcissistic features in a direction opposite to that of shame.

Gramzow and Tangney (1992) also considered measures of two related constructs: selfism and splitting. *Selfism*, one of the hallmarks of narcissism, refers to a tendency to regard most situations in an egocentric or selfish manner (Phares & Erkine, 1984)—that is, to evaluate a wide range of situations in terms of what can be gained for the self, independent of others' needs. As one might expect, selfism was positively correlated with NPI scores, particularly the more maladaptive Exploitativeness/Entitlement factor. Selfism, however, was unrelated to participants' tendency to experience shame, most likely because this egocentric aspect of narcissism is less directly relevant to shame-related issues (e.g., vulnerability of the self). The observed negative relationship between guilt and selfism is interesting in light of our findings regarding the positive link between guilt and empathy (Tangney, 1991; see Chapter 5). Guilt-prone individuals appear generally more other-oriented than self-oriented.

Kernberg (1975) identified *splitting* as a key defense of individuals with borderline and narcissistic personality disorders. Splitting is characterized by dramatic shifts in the evaluation of the self and others. In the course of everyday life, narcissists are inclined to alternate between the extremes of idealization, on the one hand, and degradation, on the other, in an attempt to avoid the conflicts and complexity of simultaneously dealing with both "good" and "bad" aspects of the self or another person. For example, narcissistic individuals are known to hold extreme views of friends and family members. On one day, they may describe a new acquaintance as "the most wonderful, brilliant, best friend one could imagine," whereas on the next day they may describe the same individual as "a hateful, deceitful, stupid lout." Although splitting is theoretically normative at early stages of development, it is generally regarded as a pathological defense among adults. In the Gramzow and Tangney (1992) study, shame-proneness was strongly positively correlated with splitting.

In sum, our findings underscore the importance of differentiating between measures of pathological and more benign types of narcissism. As Freud (1914/1957) noted, narcissistic processes are a universal component of personality development. A certain degree of self-focus and self-regard is essential to the development of a coherent personality structure. Exner (1986), for example, cautions that individuals with unusually low scores on the Rorschach Egocentricity ratio are at risk for psychological disorders, presumably because such individuals lack sufficient self-focus and self-investment. In other words, such individuals may be characterized by a deficit in "healthy" narcissism.

As discussed, the NPI appears to assess generally adaptive components of narcissism. Thus it is perhaps not surprising that shame-proneness was generally inversely related to this measure. In contrast, the clinical literature has been exclusively concerned with the dynamics of shame in connection with pathological narcissism. And in the Gramzow and Tangney (1992) study, it was only the maladaptive component of the NPI that was positively associated with the tendency to experience the ugly feeling of shame.

SUMMARY AND CONCLUSIONS

Shame and guilt are "*self*-conscious" emotions. They are intimately intertwined in our relationship with our self. On the one hand, feelings of shame and guilt arise in the context of self-blame. When we fail or transgress, we are naturally drawn to search for explanations and causes. And when the finger of blame points squarely at the self, we are likely to feel shame or guilt. Self-focused feelings of shame are especially relevant to people's self-esteem. In this chapter, we have discussed the interplay between shame and self-esteem, noting that these are related but distinct constructs. We have speculated that frequent and repeated experiences of shame are apt to "chip away" at people's general level of self-esteem. On the flip side of the coin, low self-esteem is likely to increase people's vulnerability to feelings of shame. Nonetheless, research has shown that there is not a one-to-one relationship between shame and low self-esteem. The correlation is considerable, but we speculate that there are a number of factors that moderate this link between shame-proneness and level self-esteem. We have also considered the implications of situation-specific self-awareness and related traits such as self-consciousness and self-monitoring for people's likelihood of experiencing shame and guilt. And we further explored the relevance of self beliefs and self discrepancies to these self-conscious emotions. Finally, we summarized results indicating that maladaptive aspects of narcissism are related to the egocentric experience of shame but not the behavior-focused experience of guilt.

NOTES

1. In this regard, proneness to shame bears some resemblance to the construct of (in)stability of self-esteem (Kernis, Grannemann, & Barclay, 1989; M. Rosenberg, 1965), the degree to which a person's level of self-esteem fluctuates from day to day or moment to moment. And, in fact, shame-proneness, as assessed by the SCAAI and TOSCA, is inversely correlated with Stability of Self-Esteem, as assessed by Rosenberg's (1965) scale (across seven studies of undergraduates, the mean r is $-.34$). From a conceptual standpoint, however, shame-proneness represents a tendency to experience sudden drops in self-regard *in conjunction with* the complex array of affective, cognitive and motivational features that comprise feelings of shame.

2. As discussed in Chapter 3, several theorists have introduced the notion of "internalized shame" (Cook, 1988; Kaufman, 1985, 1989) defined as an "enduring, chronic shame that has become internalized as part of one's identity and which can be most succinctly characterized as a deep sense of inferiority, inadequacy, or deficiency" (Cook, 1988). The construct of "internalized shame" treads dangerously close to the construct of self-esteem. And, in fact, Cook (1988, 1991) reports extremely high correlations (generally about $-.80$) between his Internalized Shame Scale (ISS) and traditional measures of self-esteem. Thus, there appear to be serious problems with the discriminant validity of this "internalized shame" construct and associated measures.

3. For example in three independent studies of undergraduates ($n = 249$, $n = 264$, $n = 86$), we have found correlations of .24, .29, and .29, respectively, between public self-consciousness and shame. In contrast there was no significant relationship between guilt and public self-consciousness (correlations ranged from .00 to .09). The relationship of private self-consciousness to both shame and guilt was modest at best, correlations ranging from .03 to .15 across the three studies. Similar results were reported by Davrill, Johnson, and Danko (1992).

4. An additional study of 86 undergraduates yielded similar results, although the correlation between guilt-proneness and self-monitoring was not significant.

5. In addition, we found no evidence to support the more general proposition that specific self-discrepancies are differentially related to distinct emotion symptoms or experiences (e.g., dejection vs. agitation-related experiences). Rather, self-discrepancies were related to emotional distress across the board (e.g., shame, depression, anxiety). There was no discernible difference among the specific self-discrepancies in terms of their emotion/symptom correlates.

Chapter 5

MORAL EMOTIONS AND INTERPERSONAL SENSITIVITY

Empathy Enters the Picture

> I am often impressed with the fact that even a minimal
> amount of empathic understanding—a bumbling and faulty
> attempt to catch the confused complexity of the client's
> meaning—is helpful, though there is no doubt that it is most
> helpful when I can see and formulate clearly the meanings in
> his experiencing which for him have been unclear and
> tangled.
>
> —ROGERS (1961, pp. 53–54)

In this chapter, we shift from a focus on the self to our interactions with others. Thus far, we have been discussing the implications of shame and guilt for self-relevant experiences. We now turn our attention outward, to the implications of shame and guilt for our interpersonal relationships. And, in this chapter, we focus specifically on empathy and empathy-related processes as they relate to shame and guilt.

EMPATHY: THE "GOOD" MORAL AFFECTIVE CAPACITY

Famed clinical psychologist and leader of the humanistic school of psychotherapy, Carl R. Rogers (1961) recognized that empathy is a fundamental component of close, mutually rewarding relationships. Subsequent research has certainly supported this notion. There is vast empirical literature indicating that empathy facilitates altruistic, helping behavior (Eisenberg, 1986, 2000; Eisenberg et al., 1996; Feshbach, 1975b, 1978, 1987; Feshbach & Feshbach, 1986; for a review, see Eisenberg & Miller, 1987), that it fosters warm, close interpersonal relationships, and that it inhibits interpersonal aggression (Eisenberg, 1986; Feshbach, 1975b, 1984, 1987; Feshbach & Feshbach, 1969, 1982, 1986; Saarni, 1999; for a review, see P. A. Miller & Eisenberg, 1988). The empathic component of helping behaviors begins early in life. For example, Eisenberg-Berg and Neal (1979) demonstrated that when 4- and 5-year-old preschoolers explained why they had performed a prosocial act, they most often referred to the needs of another as the motivating factor.

Empathy has also been identified as an essential component of numerous valued social processes, including positive parent–child relationships (Feshbach, 1987), effective client–therapist interactions (Rogers, 1975), and individuals' application of moral principles to real-life interpersonal situations (Eisenberg, 2000; Hoffman, 1987; Saarni, 1999).

Thus, empathy is the "good" moral affective capacity or experience, leading us in moral directions and diverting us from paths of vice and perdition. Experiences of empathy help us to accurately "read" or interpret interpersonal events, allowing us to respond sensitively to the feelings of others. Perhaps most important, empathy helps us recognize when our actions adversely affect others and it motivates us to take corrective steps to remedy the situation.

VARIATIONS ON A THEME:
EMPATHY, SYMPATHY, AND PERSONAL DISTRESS

The *American Heritage Dictionary* defines empathy as "understanding so intimate that the feelings, thoughts, and motives of one are readily comprehended by another." Psychologists have devoted a good deal of attention to the development and implications of empathy, and we now have a fairly extensive theoretical and empirical literature related to the construct of empathy. Early formulations of empathy tended to emphasize either the cognitive or affective components of empathy, whereas more recent theories acknowledge and integrate both cognitive and affective components of empathic responsiveness (M. H. Davis, 1980, 1983; Feshbach, 1975a).

UCLA psychologist Norma D. Feshbach (1975a), for example, defines empathy as a "shared emotional response between an observer and a stimulus person." She suggests that empathic responsiveness requires three interrelated skills or capacities: (1) the cognitive ability to take another person's perspective, (2) the cognitive ability to accurately recognize and discriminate another person's affective experience, and (3) the affective ability to personally experience a range of emotions (since empathy involves sharing another person's emotional experience). Similarly, Coke, Batson, and McDavis (1978) proposed a two-stage model of empathic responding including both cognitive and affective components. In this model, perspective taking facilitates empathic concern and, in turn, empathic concern results in a desire to help. M. H. Davis (1980) expanded on this idea by emphasizing a multidimensional approach to measuring empathy, also emphasizing both cognitive and affective components of empathy.

Some researchers have made a distinction between empathy and sympathy. Eisenberg (1986) explains that sympathy involves feelings of *concern* for the situation or emotional state of another but does not necessarily involve the vicarious experience of the other person's feelings or emotions (e.g., emotional matching). Thus, one may feel concern (sympathy) for an angered individual without being vicariously angered oneself (an empathic reaction).

An even more critical distinction has been made between "other-oriented" empathy and "self-oriented" personal distress (Batson, 1990; Batson & Coke, 1981; M. H. Davis, 1983; Fultz, Batson, Fortenbach, McCarthy, & Varney, 1986). With other-oriented empathic responses, the observer is able to take the other person's perspective, and vicariously experience similar feelings. These responses often involve feelings of sympathy and concern for the other person, and often lead to extending aid or comfort to the distressed other. Most importantly, the empathic individual's focus remains on the experiences and needs of the *other person*, not on his or her own empathic response. Alternatively, self-oriented personal distress involves a primary focus on the feelings, needs, and experiences of the *empathizer*. As M. H. Davis (1983) demonstrated, personal distress is a distinct subset of empathy that is strongly associated with vulnerability, uncertainty, and fearfulness.

Several empirical studies have underscored the importance of this distinction between other-oriented empathy and self-oriented personal

distress. Empathic concern for others has been linked to altruistic helping behavior, whereas self-oriented personal distress is unrelated to altruism (Batson et al., 1988). Similarly, M. H. Davis and Oathout (1987)
found that among romantic couples, personal distress was associated
with negative interpersonal behaviors. In addition, personal distress has
been demonstrated to interfere with prosocial behaviors in both children (Eisenberg, Fabes, Carlo, et al., 1993; Eisenberg, Fabes, Miller, et
al., 1990) and adolescents (Estrada, 1995).

In sum, current conceptualizations of empathy integrate both affective and cognitive components. Empathy involves both cognitive perspective taking and the affective ability to vicariously experience a
range of emotions. Some researchers have highlighted the distinction
between "true" empathy (involving an affective "match") and sympathy
(feelings of concern without a shared emotional experience). Others
have made the critical distinction between other-oriented empathy and
self-oriented personal distress. This latter distinction seems especially
important in that personal distress reactions, which shift the focus away
from others, can actually have a detrimental effect on interpersonal relationships.

MORAL AFFECT: THE GOOD, THE BAD, AND THE UGLY

Together with empathy, shame and guilt are generally regarded as
"moral" emotions that help us "keep to the straight and narrow." Like
empathy, shame and guilt (or the anticipation of these emotions) are
presumed to inhibit all manner of misdeeds and wrongdoing. And, just
as understanding another's distress (i.e., empathy) serves to motivate
reparative action, shame and guilt are thought to foster repair—
confession, apology, atonement.

A question that naturally arises is "How do these moral affective
processes work together?" One might expect shame, guilt, and empathy
to work hand in hand, leading us down the moral path, avoiding sinful
acts. Recent research, however, indicates that although guilt and empathy may work together in a mutually enhancing fashion, shame can
actually interfere with an other-oriented empathic connection.

Consider first people's interpersonal focus when they are experiencing shame versus guilt. Several years ago, we asked several hundred
children and adults to describe a recent personal experience of shame
and guilt (Tangney et al., 1994), and we later coded these accounts

along a number of dimensions. One area of interest concerned people's interpersonal focus when describing these personal shame and guilt experiences. Here we found systematic differences in the nature of respondents' interpersonal concerns as they described their personal failures, misdeeds, and transgressions. The shame experiences reported by adults were especially likely to involve a concern with others' evaluations of the self. On the other hand, guilt experiences were more likely to involve a concern with one's effect on others. This difference in "egocentric" versus "other-oriented" concerns isn't surprising, given that shame involves a focus on the self whereas guilt relates to a specific behavior. A shamed person who is focusing on negative *self*-evaluations would naturally be drawn to a concern over others' evaluations. It's a short leap from thinking what a horrible person you are to thinking about how *others* might be evaluating you. In contrast, a person experiencing guilt is already relatively "decentered"—focusing on a negative *behavior* somewhat separate from the self. In focusing on a bad behavior, rather than a bad self, a person in the midst of a guilt experience is more likely to recognize (and have concerns about) the effects of that behavior *on others* rather than on others' evaluations of the self.

And, indeed, when people describe guilt-inducing events, they convey more other-oriented empathy than when they describe shame-inducing events. For example, in the same study of children and adults, we also coded participants' shame and guilt narratives for markers of other-oriented concern and interpersonal empathy specifically. As you might expect, people expressed more empathy for others involved in guilt episodes compared to shame episodes (Tangney et al., 1994), consistent with the notion that there is a special link between guilt and empathy (e.g., Eisenberg, 1986; Hoffman, 1982; Zahn-Waxler & Robinson, 1995). By its very nature, guilt forms a bridge to other-oriented empathic concern (Tangney, 1991, 1995b). In focusing on an offending behavior, the person experiencing guilt is relatively free of the egocentric, self-involved process characteristic of shame. In fact, this focus on a specific behavior is likely to highlight the consequences of that behavior for a distressed other. In this way, guilt serves to foster an other-oriented empathic connection.

For example, 25-year-old Tina recounted this guilt experience:

> "I remember feeling very guilty for being so angry at my father over a particular fight. In fact, I still feel guilty today, as I see him getting older and weaker, over all the fights we ever had. The conflict here is

this: He is a very strict man, a military man, and raised me extremely harshly. He infuriated me so much that I would become defensive. I learned to fend for my beliefs and my rights. If I hadn't, I would have become a submissive fool. The guilt comes when I realize that he would do anything for me. He only tried his best, even though it wasn't right. I feel bad for all the hurt I've caused him, because of his sternness."

The link between guilt and empathy is evident among children as well. For example, 8-year-old Susie recounted this recent guilt experience:

"Well, I was at this camp in music. We were playing elimination freeze tag. The music stops and you freeze. I was right on Jessica, and I lost my balance and she had to go out because she moved. [How were you feeling?] Sad and mad at myself. [What were you thinking?] Darn, why did I hit her? Why did I mess her up? She didn't deserve to get out—I did."

In contrast to the apparently synergistic effect between guilt and empathy, there is reason to suspect that feelings of shame may actually interfere with empathic responsiveness. Shame is an acutely painful experience, involving a marked self-focus that is incompatible with other-oriented empathy reactions (Tangney, 1991, 1995b). The tremendous preoccupation with the self draws one's focus away from a distressed other, thus short-circuiting other-oriented feelings of empathy. In effect, shamed individuals are less likely to be concerned with the pain experienced by the harmed other and are more consumed with a focus on negative characteristics of the self: *I* am such a horrible person (for having hurt so-and-so). In fact, rather than promoting other-oriented empathic concern, the acute self-focus of shame is likely to foster self-oriented personal distress responses. Hoffman (1984) has noted that empathy is sometimes derailed by an *egoistic drift* whereby a self-focused person's empathic focus on another person is interrupted when the empathic affect resonates with the observer's own needs. From this perspective, it seems likely that shame brings a person one step closer to a personal distress reaction and several steps further from true other-oriented empathy.

For example, 20-year-old Pat described this shame-inducing situation:

"I was sitting with a group of friends, one of whom was telling jokes. He started telling very rude racist jokes (about blacks, putting them down). Although I realized this was inappropriate, I did not make the effort to tell the person and was eventually taken in by the jokes. I did not realize that a friend of mine who is black and with whom I participated in a 'racism workshop' was sitting at the table directly behind us and had heard every single word. When I noticed her, I felt the greatest shame."

When asked what he was feeling and thinking and what he did, Pat responded:

"The feeling was unbearable—guilt and shame—thinking of what she must think of me and that I deserve it. I hated myself . . . I just said hello to the person (the black friend) and said nothing more . . . I most likely blushed. I must have looked shocked at seeing her. I left alone—not with the group."

When asked how the other person reacted, Pat indicated:

"She didn't say anything, I guess pretended like she didn't hear (just so she wouldn't embarrass me!)."

Pat obviously had a very strong emotional reaction to this event, but his reaction was solidly self-focused. Note that there was no mention of how his black friend might have felt upon hearing the racist jokes—no notion that *the friend* might have been hurt or distressed by the event. Instead Pat's focus is on *Pat*—not only on how Pat felt about himself, but also on how the black friend might be evaluating Pat. Pat is so wrapped up in his feelings of shame that he is, for the moment at least, incapable of taking his friend's perspective except as it relates to feelings about Pat. In short, this vignette illustrates how the acute self-focus of shame can interfere with a true other-oriented empathic response.

The notion that guilt and empathy may work hand in hand whereas shame may disrupt an empathic connection was further supported by Leith and Baumeister (1998). In two studies, undergraduate participants were asked to describe the most intense interpersonal conflict they had experienced in the past 6 months, first from their own perspective and then from their partner's perspective. Leith and Baumeister (1998) coded markers of shame and guilt in the initial description, and examined the degree to which shame and guilt were associated with the participant's ability to shift perspective (i.e., provide new or different information when describing the event from the other person's point of view). In both studies, shifts in perspective taking were associated with more prevalent guilt-related themes in the initial description of the conflict event. In other words, it appeared that people who experienced guilt were better able to put themselves in the other person's shoes. Experiences of shame were less consistently related to shifts in perspective taking. However, when significant, shame was associated with impaired perspective taking.

It's worth noting again that this inhibition or interruption of empathy is not a trivial matter. A great deal of research has shown that empathy is a key element in facilitating positive interactions with others (e.g., Eisenberg & Miller, 1987; Feshbach, 1987; P. A. Miller & Eisenberg, 1988). Not surprisingly, in Leith and Baumeister's (1998) studies, guilt was associated with positive relationship outcomes; in contrast, shame was more likely to be associated with deterioration or dissolution of the relationship in question.

DISPOSITIONAL TENDENCIES TO EXPERIENCE SHAME, GUILT, AND EMPATHY

Thus far, we have been focusing on situation-specific episodes of shame and guilt, examining markers of other-oriented empathy *in specific situations*. The studies we have described so far speak to the experiences and responses of the "average person on the streets." What happens when you, or I, or our neighbor next door, experiences an episode of shame or guilt? How do these emotions affect our likelihood of feeling empathy for the other people involved in a particular event? Studies of shame and guilt "states" indicate that feelings of guilt "in the moment" foster an empathic response whereas feelings of shame "in the moment" interfere with an other-oriented empathic connection.

We've also examined the interrelationship of shame, guilt, and empathy at the level of *dispositions*. Most people experience shame, guilt, and empathy at various points in their lives; that is, people have the capacity to experience each of the emotional reactions. But there are also *individual differences* in the degree to which people are "prone" to particular kinds of emotional events. Just as people vary in their "proneness" to experience shame or guilt across a variety of situations in day-to-day life, people vary in their capacity to respond empathically to others. Some people are more empathic than the average person; other people are less empathic. How do shame-prone and guilt-prone dispositions relate to dispositional empathy? As you might guess, the differential link of shame and guilt to empathy observed in specific situations is also evident in studies of moral affective dispositions. Across numerous independent studies, our findings indicate that the shame-prone person is not an empathic person. That is, individual differences in proneness to shame are inversely related to a dispositional capacity for empathy; conversely, proneness to guilt is positively correlated with empathic responsiveness (Tangney, 1991, 1994, 1995a, 1995b, 1995c; Tangney, Wagner, Burggraf, Gramzow, & Fletcher, 1991). (Table A.3 in Appendix A shows the results from 11 independent studies, including data from children, adolescents, college students, and adults from many walks of life.)

To assess individual differences in adult empathy, we most often have used M. H. Davis's (1983) 28-item Interpersonal Reactivity Index (IRI), which explicitly distinguishes between other-oriented empathy and self-oriented personal distress. The Perspective Taking Scale assesses the ability to "step outside of the self" and take another's perspective in real-life situations. Most researchers regard perspective-taking as the quintessential component of other-oriented empathy. The Fantasy Scale assesses perspective-taking in the fictional realm (e.g., identifying with the feelings of a character in a book). The Empathic Concern Scale assesses the extent to which respondents experience "other-oriented" feelings of compassion and concern. And, of special interest, the Personal Distress Scale assesses the degree to which respondents experience "self-oriented" discomfort or fear when faced with another's distress. The Personal Distress Scale taps empathic overconcern, and there is also an element of "loss of control" inherent in many of the items.

We've also used Feshbach and Lipian's (1987) Empathy Scale for Adults, Lipian and Feshbach's (1987) Empathy Scale for Children, and Feshbach and Caskey's (1987) Parent/Partner Empathy Scale. Each of the Feshbach measures focus primarily on a capacity for other-oriented empathy. The 59-item Empathy Scale for Adults (Feshbach & Lipian, 1987) yields four empathy subscales and a combined Total Empathy Index. Three of the subscales assess the three components of empathy described by Feshbach (1975a): Cognitive Empathy (role taking, perspective taking—e.g., "I try to see things through the eyes of others");

Affective Cue Discrimination (the ability to perceive others' affective states accurately—e.g., "I pick up changes in other people's moods that most others miss"); and Emotional Responsiveness (the ability to experience a range of affect—e.g., "I find it difficult to hold back tears at weddings"). A fourth subscale, General Empathy, assesses a general capacity for empathic response, which is theoretically dependent on each of the three components described above (e.g., "I get very involved in the stories people tell me" and "It hurts me to see someone I know in pain").

Taken together, our findings strongly support the hypothesized link between guilt and other-oriented empathy. For example, across eight independent studies employing the IRI, proneness to "shame-free" guilt (i.e., the guilt residuals) was positively and consistently related to Perspective Taking and Empathic Concern. In each case, these correlations were substantial and statistically significant. Similarly, across four studies using Feshbach and Lipian's (1987) Empathy Scale for Adults, guilt was positively correlated with empathy.

Results involving proneness to shame showed a very different pattern of results. Proneness to shame was negatively or negligibly related to other-oriented empathy and positively related to personal distress. The inverse relationship between shame and empathy is most evident in studies employing Feshbach and colleagues' measures, particularly when Cognitive Empathy and Affective Cue Recognition are considered. Similarly, in a study of parents and grandparents of fifth-grade children (Tangney, Wagner, & Barlow, 2001), indices of other-oriented empathy were consistently positively correlated with guilt and negatively correlated with shame across these various subsamples. (Parents and grandparents in this study completed Feshbach & Caskey's [1987] Parent/Partner Empathy Scale.)

As already noted, the distinction between other-oriented empathy and self-oriented personal distress is of special interest when researchers are considering shame and guilt. We predicted that whereas guilt should be related to other-oriented empathy, shame should be much more closely associated with self-oriented personal distress responses. The M. H. Davis (1983) IRI measure of empathy is unique in providing an explicit means of differentiating between components of other-oriented empathy and those of personal distress. And, in fact, we observed a strong positive link between proneness to shame and self-oriented personal distress responses, consistent across studies. Among adults from many different walks of life, shame-prone individuals appear more vulnerable to an "egoistic drift" when faced with distressed others. They are more inclined to be sidetracked by their own emotional response, rather than remaining focused on the other person's feelings and needs.

We have also examined the relationship of shame and guilt to empathy in a substantial sample of children and adolescents. As in the college and adult samples, proneness to guilt was clearly related to a capacity for empathy, but so too was shame-proneness. Given that both studies employed the same short measure of empathy by Lipian and Feshbach (1987), it is unclear whether this pattern reflects limitations of that single brief measure, or a bona fide developmental shift in the implications of shame for other-oriented empathy.

AN EXPERIMENTAL STUDY:
EFFECTS OF INDUCED SHAME ON EMPATHY

Finally, in our laboratory we have begun a series of studies where we experimentally induce feelings of shame in participants randomly assigned to a "shame condition" and then examine the effects of the shame induction on empathy, altruism, covert aggression, and so forth. The first of these studies focused on the link between shame and empathy (Marschall, 1996). Marschall induced feelings of shame by providing participants with false negative feedback on a purported intelligence test. After making a fairly public estimate of their test scores, participants in the shame condition were told they scored substantially below their guess by an experimenter who exchanged shocked, surprised, and then dubious expressions with an assistant. A postmanipulation check, using the State Shame and Guilt Scale (SSGS; Marschall et al., 1994; see Chapter 3) showed that participants in the "shame" condition experienced significantly more feelings of shame than did participants receiving neutral feedback. (The experiment was immediately followed with extensive "process" debriefing procedures, conducted by carefully trained and closely supervised senior research assistants.)

Marschall found that people induced to feel shame subsequently reported less empathy for a disabled student in an apparently unrelated task immediately following the above procedure. Interestingly, this effect was particularly pronounced among low-shame-prone individuals. Consistent with results from our dispositional studies (Tangney, 1991, 1995b), shame-prone individuals are pretty unempathic across the board, regardless of whether they are shamed in the laboratory or not.

But among their less shame-prone peers—who show a fair capacity for empathy in general—the shame induction appears to "short-circuit" participants' empathic responsiveness. In short, as a result of the shame induction, low-shame-prone people were rendered relatively unempathic—more like their shame-prone peers.

SUMMARY AND CONCLUSIONS

This chapter examined how various moral affective processes work together. In addition to shame and guilt, empathy is an important moral affective guide. Researchers and clinicians alike would readily agree that the capacity for empathy facilitates positive, mutually rewarding interpersonal relationships. Further, empathy inhibits aversive and destructive behaviors toward others. We have summarized a wide range of studies that demonstrate a strong positive link between guilt and empathy at the level of both situations and dispositions. Guilt and empathy appear to work hand in hand in a mutually enhancing fashion. In contrast, there are numerous empirical indications that feelings of shame actually interfere with other-oriented empathic responses. Rather, shame appears to set the stage for self-oriented personal distress reactions, where the individual's focus on a distressed other is "derailed" by his or her own emotional experience. These relationships are not only supported by real-life narratives of specific shame and guilt events but are also readily apparent in correlational studies of moral affective dispositions, as well as in an experimental study involving shame inductions. Thus, in this chapter, guilt along with empathy emerge as a "good" moral affective experience. On the other hand, we have seen yet another indication of the dark side of shame—in this case, in the realm of interpersonal relationships. And this is just the beginning of the story. Next, in Chapter 6, we describe research showing that at times shame can turn downright nasty!

Chapter 6

SHAMED INTO ANGER?

The Special Link between Shame and Interpersonal Hostility

Creeping up my throat like a scarlet plague
The bile of my anger and shame overtakes me
My arm longs to lash out with a tigress' claws
To hurt, to maim, to inflict, to make bleed
All those who taunt me.
                          —ANONYMOUS (1993)

In this chapter, we examine the implications of shame and guilt for the experience and expression of anger. It is often assumed that, as "moral emotions," shame and guilt help people curb socially unacceptable impulses such as anger and aggression. We assumed that, too, when we first began our research on shame and guilt. We just assumed that anger would be inversely related to shame and guilt. It seemed reasonable that both shame and guilt experiences would make one less likely to lash out toward another person in an angry or aggressive manner. We took it for granted that, upon experiencing guilt, an individual would focus on the act and would subsequently focus on reparative actions or alternative actions for the future. Similarly, we thought that a shamed person would be so focused on his or her "bad self," turning blame inward, that the question of others' blame would be moot. He or she would thus be unlikely to experience anger directed toward others. Furthermore, one could reason that for the person well acquainted with shame, just the risk of a shame reaction would inhibit anger and aggression.

SHAME, BLAME, AND ANGER: SOME EARLY CLUES

By chance, we caught an initial glimpse of the dynamics among shame, guilt, and anger when we looked at the correlates of externalization responses on the SCAAI. As discussed in Chapter 3, both the SCAAI and TOSCA measures include, in addition to shame and guilt responses, items assessing externalization of blame. Externalization of blame involves attribution of cause to external factors, to aspects of the situation, or to another person. For example, in the TOSCA-A, our adolescent measure, we ask participants to imagine the following: "You trip in the cafeteria and spill your friend's drink." The externalization response to this scenario is "I would think: 'I couldn't help it. The floor was slippery.' "

We assumed—and attribution theory would strongly suggest—a negative relationship between externalization and both shame and guilt. After all, externalization involves an external attribution whereas shame and guilt are related to internal or self-attributions. What we found, however, was a strong positive relationship between externalization and shame, on the one hand, and negative or negligible correlations between externalization and shame-free guilt, on the other. At first, we were puzzled. We entertained the possibility that we had miscoded one of the variables. But then, as it became clear that this was a bona fide result, replicating across study after study, it began to make sense.

THE DYNAMICS OF THE SHAME-TO-ANGER LINK

As early as 1971, Helen Block Lewis proposed that there is an intrinsic link between shame and anger. She suggested that although a shamed individual's hostility is initially directed inward, toward the self, the experience is so aversive that there is often an inclination to shift that hostility and blame outward (see also Retzinger, 1987; Scheff, 1987). As indicated earlier, shame can be an extremely painful and devastating emotion. When people feel shame over a particular failure or transgression, they are berating themselves not just for the specific event; rather, they are damning *themselves*—the core of their being—as flawed, useless, despicable. In this way, shame experiences pose a tremendous threat to the self. Lewis (1971) suggests that the feeling of shame evokes such strong feelings of anger and hostility toward the self that the individual may feel "overwhelmed and paralyzed" (p. 41) by it.

To make matters even worse, there are very few options for remediating the problem posed by shame. Efforts to change one's future behavior, acts of contrition, attempts to fix or otherwise compensate for the harmful consequences of the specific event—such corrective measures don't quite do it. In fact, these efforts at remediation miss the whole point because the shamed individual is still stuck with the problem of a hopelessly defective self. And, of course, a shamed person can't change fundamental aspects of the self overnight. So there he or she is—hopelessly mired in an agonizing, ego-threatening state of shame with no obvious way out.

How do people, in the midst of a shame experience, attempt to cope with or contain this hateful emotion? As discussed in Chapter 4, little research has examined people's strategies for diffusing feelings of shame and guilt, but we speculate that there are at least two obvious paths that a shamed individual might take.

One option is to withdraw—escaping the shame-inducing situation and hiding the horrible self from the view of others. Research has consistently shown that feelings of shame are often associated with a desire to hide or escape (Barrett et al., 1993; H. B. Lewis, 1971; Lindsay-Hartz, 1984; Tangney, 1993b; Tangney, Miller, & Flicker, 1992). The withdrawal strategy, however, is apt to be only partially effective. In reality, the shamed, withdrawn individual is still saddled with a loathsome self. When it comes to a shamed self, there is some truth to the notion that "You can run but you can't hide!"

Another possible coping strategy—and one more likely to be effective, at least in the short run—is to turn the tables and shift the blame outward. Blaming *others* (instead of the self) can serve an ego-protective function. A shamed person may find it much less objectionable to think, "The problem is *you*, not me! You're the lout, not me!" By externalizing blame in this way, the previously shamed individual attempts to defend and preserve his or her self-esteem.

For example, 21-year-old Lisa described this shame experience:

"When I was in high school, I used to sometimes steal change from my mother's purse. Finally, I got caught—for stealing a quarter. The worst part about it was that they had suspected all along but didn't want to believe I would steal from them. *I felt awful, very ashamed, but also very angry and rebellious.* I didn't want to admit to myself that I had been doing something wrong, *because I didn't want to think of myself as a bad person.*" [emphasis added]

As a bonus, such externalized blame can serve to reduce painful self-awareness. Previous research has shown that induced states of self-awareness are often uncomfortable, if not downright aversive, particularly when negative aspects of the self have been primed or highlighted (D. Davis & Brock, 1975; Gibbons & Wicklund, 1982; Ickes, Wicklund, & Ferris, 1973). If ever there was a case of negative self-awareness, shame is it! Here's a situation in which people would be especially motivated to shift focus—to reduce self-awareness by turning the tables and shifting the blame outward!

And as a further bonus, the accompanying feelings of self-righteous anger can help the shamed person to regain some sense of agency and control. Anger is an emotion of potency and authority. In contrast, shame is an emotion of the worthless, the paralyzed, the ineffective. Thus, by redirecting hostility, by turning their anger outward, shamed individuals become angry instead, reactivating and bolstering the self, which was previously so impaired by the shame experience.

In short, the shame-to-anger defense may be quite compelling to shamed individuals. And there are two additional factors that further facilitate the shift from shame to anger: imagery of a "disapproving other," and the impaired capacity for empathy that accompanies shame.

Shame is an emotion of self-blame, involving negative evaluations of the global self. But the shame experience also evokes an image of a disapproving other. Although shame is not more public than guilt in terms of the actual structure of the emotion-eliciting experience (both emotions are typically experienced in interpersonal contexts; see Chapter 2), shamed individuals have a heightened awareness of and concern with others' evaluations. A shamed person is acutely conscious of what other people might be thinking about them. From there, it's a short step to attribute the *cause* of painful shame feelings to others who are perceived as disapproving. Like guilt, shame events typically occur in interpersonal contexts, so attributions for the negative emotions can be readily directed toward others involved in the interaction. Feeling shamed, feeling diminished in comparison to others, and simultaneously scrutinized and *evaluated* by others, it's relatively easy to blame the painful experience of shame on the observer. (Notice that the observing other may or may not be engaging in such negative evaluation of the shamed person. The point is that the phenomenology of shame itself involves a heightened awareness of others' presumed evaluations.)

Moreover, shamed people are apt to feel they are getting a raw deal from those perceived "disapproving others" who have ostensibly caused their experience of shame. After all, they only made one mistake, one transgression, one sin. Suddenly their entire self is being negatively evaluated. It feels unfair! In fact, one could become downright angry! "How could they treat me like this!" In this way, the imagery of a disapproving other may contribute to the shift from shame to outwardly directed anger.

Finally, as described in greater detail in Chapter 5, feelings of shame seem to interfere with people's ability to empathize with others. Thus, shamed people are less inclined toward empathy—empathy that might otherwise help curb their tendency to externalize blame and lash out in anger.

SHAME-FUELED ANGER: RELATIONSHIP IMPLICATIONS

It almost goes without saying that such shame-based anger can pose serious problems for our interpersonal relationships. The recipients of shame-motivated anger are apt to experience such anger as erupting "out of the blue." Feeling that it makes little rational sense, the hapless observing other is often left wondering, "Where did *that* come from?!"

For example, Brad, a 42 year-old executive shared this shame experience:

"I did something I knew was wrong and a friend confronted me. *I wanted to blame him* for the awkwardness of the situation . . . even though I knew I was at fault." [emphasis added]

Although we don't know the exact nature of Brad's transgression, clearly he knew at heart that he was wrong, he wanted to blame his friend "for the awkwardness of the situation" (which we read as "the painfulness of the situation"). What is notable in this account, and in other similar accounts from our studies, is that this sort of shame-induced defensive externalization is fairly irrational, even from the perspective of the shamed individual. No doubt, the recipient of such shame-induced anger may also experience such exchanges as unjustified and irrational. For example, Brad's friend may well have been dumbfounded by Brad's off-the-wall implication of blame. Depending on the context and the depth of the friendship, this sort of inexplicable exchange may mark a serious turning point in a relationship.

Thus, although defensive anger may represent a short-term gain in lessening the pain of shame in the moment, on balance this sort of shame-blame sequence is likely to be destructive for interpersonal relationships—both in the moment and in the long run. Defensive shame-based blame and anger may subsequently lead either to withdrawal (by either party or both parties) or to escalating antagonism, blame, and counterblame. In either case, the end result is likely to be a rift in the interpersonal relationship.

GUILT AND ANGER DO NOT GO HAND IN HAND

As we have discussed, feelings of guilt are typically less painful and less ego-threatening than negative feelings of shame about the self. Because the object of concern is a specific behavior, not the global self, guilt presents a much more reparable situation. Thus, we might anticipate that feelings of guilt would be less likely to invoke defensive responses, including externalization of blame, anger, and aggression. And in several other respects, too, guilt is not conducive to anger in the same way that shame is. First, the experience of guilt appears to facilitate rather than inhibit feelings of other-oriented empathy (see Chapter 5), and there is a vast literature showing that empathy is apt to curb reactions of anger and aggression (e.g., Eisenberg, 1986; Feshbach, 1975b, 1984, 1987; Feshbach & Feshbach, 1969, 1982, 1986; P. A. Miller & Eisenberg, 1988). Second, in contrast to shame, the experience of guilt is less likely to involve a concern with others' critical evaluations of the self. In fact, as described in Chapter 5, people in the midst of a guilt experience are more concerned with their effect on others. Thus, people feeling guilt are less likely to hold others responsible for their discomfort. They are less apt to perceive others as unfairly evaluating and criticizing them. And thus they are less apt to retaliate in anger against "observing others." Finally, in guilt the self is less "impaired" than in shame. Feelings of shame, not guilt, are associated with a sense of worthlessness, powerlessness, and a lack of control. Thus, people in the midst of a guilt experience may be less motivated to regain a sense of agency and control through externalization of blame and anger.

EMPIRICAL STUDIES OF SHAME, GUILT, AND ANGER

Thus far, we have provided a conceptual discussion of the hypothesized dynamics between shame and anger. We have suggested that, for a variety of reasons, feelings of shame are apt to invoke defensive reactions including externalization of blame and anger. In contrast, we have speculated that feelings of guilt (about specific behaviors) are less likely to provoke an angry defensive response. What do the data actually show?

As discussed earlier, our initial studies employing the SCAAI and TOSCA measures indicated strong and consistent positive correlations between shame-proneness and externalization of blame. In contrast, the tendency to experience "shame-free" guilt was negligibly or negatively related to externalization of blame. In short, when faced with a failure or transgression, people who are inclined to feel shame about the self also show the tendency to blame *others* for such negative events. In contrast, guilt-prone people are apt to accept responsibility, feeling bad about the behavior and owning their role in the situation. Moreover, this pattern of results has been evident in each and every study we have conducted—with children, with adolescents, with college students, with adults of all ages, with people from diverse backgrounds and walks of life (for a table of representative results, see Tangney, 1994).

The results involving externalization of blame are consistent with the notion of a link between shame and anger, but the SCAAI and TOSCA externalization scales assess a cognitive attributional dimension (externalization of blame), not affective anger per se. In a series of subsequent studies, we examined the relationship of shame and guilt to anger more directly by including more mainstream measures of anger arousal and hostility. The findings from these studies converged neatly with the externalization results (Tangney, Wagner, Fletcher, & Gramzow, 1992; Tangney, 1993a, 1994, 1995a, 1995b, 1995c). For example, in three independent samples ($n = 243$, $n = 188$, and $n = 252$), college students completed the Trait Anger Scale (TAS; Spielberger, Gorsuch, & Lushene, 1970) and the SCAAI and/or TOSCA. Across all studies, proneness to shame was significantly positively correlated with TAS Trait Anger. In Studies 1 and 3 we also administered the Symptom

Checklist 90 (SCL-90; Derogatis, Lipman, & Covi, 1973), and in Studies 2 and 3 participants completed the Buss–Durkee Hostility Inventory (Buss & Durkee, 1957). The results were remarkably consistent across studies and measurement methods. The tendency to experience ugly feelings of shame was significantly positively correlated with SCL-90 Anger–Hostility and Paranoid Ideation subscales, as well as Buss–Durkee measures of indirect hostility, irritability, resentment, and suspicion. In contrast, proneness to "shame-free" guilt (i.e., guilt independent of the variance shared with shame) was negatively or negligibly correlated with these indices of anger and hostility. Similar findings linking shame to hostility and anger have been reported by Hoglund and Nicholas (1995).

A similar pattern was observed in a sample of 363 fifth-grade children (Tangney, Wagner, Burggraf, et al., 1991). Children completed the Children's Inventory of Anger (CIA; Finch, Saylor, & Nelson, 1987) and the TOSCA-C. Their teachers completed the teacher version of the Child Behavior Checklist (CBCL; Achenbach & Edelbrock, 1986). Among the fifth-grade males, shame-proneness was positively correlated with both self-reports of anger and teacher reports of aggression whereas guilt-proneness was negatively correlated with self-reports of anger. Among the fifth-grade females, shame-proneness was also positively correlated with self-reports of anger but unrelated to teacher reports of aggression; in contrast, there was no relationship between females' guilt-proneness and indices of anger and aggression.

In sum, both theory and research suggest that shame may not only motivate avoidant behavior (see Chapter 2)—shame can also motivate defensive feelings of anger and hostility, and a tendency to project blame outward. In contrast, guilt has been associated with a tendency to accept responsibility and, if anything, with a somewhat decreased tendency toward interpersonal anger and hostility.

CONSTRUCTIVE VERSUS DESTRUCTIVE RESPONSES TO ANGER

Conceptualization and Assessment

So far, we have been focusing on how moral affective style (i.e., shame-proneness and guilt-proneness) is related to people's readiness to become angry. The focus has been on *feelings* of anger and hostility—internal emotional experiences. Feelings are important, but ultimately we may be more concerned with what people *do* once angered. How are these feelings transformed into action?

At this point, it may be helpful to take a bit of a detour into the literature on aggression and other forms of expressing anger. We hope that this will provide a framework enabling readers to better understand our next series of studies regarding shame, guilt, and constructive versus destructive responses to anger.

Anger is pretty much inevitable in our social world. In a typical day we have many interactions with many different people. It stands to reason that not all will go smoothly, even in the happiest of lives. On occasion, people treat us unfairly. They insult us. They loaf. They irritate and annoy us. They even sometimes threaten and attack us. Anger is a normal human emotional response that is experienced with some regularity by people of all ages. (In fact, anger is one of the earliest emotions to emerge in infancy, as indicated by the onset of facial displays of anger within the first months of life; Ekman, Friesen, & Ellsworth, 1982; Izard, 1977.)

Even so, anger has gotten a pretty bad reputation over the years. We generally think of anger as a bad emotion. Many people think they shouldn't feel anger. Some deny it. And anger is something we'd rather our loved ones not feel—especially when they're angry at us!

Psychologists, too, tend to hold anger in fairly low esteem. Most would categorize anger as a "problematic" emotion. Psychotherapists search for ways to reduce the levels of anger experienced by clients. And researchers construe anger as a negative outcome—in the same heap with anxiety, depression, and paranoid ideation (Derogatis et al., 1973).

Part of the problem is that we (both psychologists and the average guy on the street) tend to use the terms "anger" and "aggression" loosely, often interchangeably. But the distinction between anger and aggression is an important one. Anger is a negative *affective state*—an emotion that involves an attribution of blame. Aggression (verbal or physical) is a *behavioral response* aimed at causing harm or distress to another. Although it is often assumed that feelings of anger typically result in aggressive responses of one sort or another (e.g., Berkowitz, 1962, 1969), Averill's (1982) research indicates that overt aggression is by no means a dominant response to anger. He estimates that, among adults, verbal aggression occurs in no more than 30–50% of daily episodes of anger, and physical aggression is quite rare (10%). And think about it. When was the last time you saw a normal, rational adult haul off and hit someone in anger? It's an unusual event!

Thus, although anger is probably a component of most aggressive incidents, most angry episodes do not involve subsequent aggressive behaviors. In Averill's (1982) studies, adults referred to a range of nonaggressive behaviors and "cognitive reappraisals" of the anger-eliciting situation in their descriptions of recent personal episodes of anger. In fact, nonaggressive "constructive" responses (e.g., rationally discussing the matter with the target of the anger) were about as common as verbal and indirect aggressive responses (e.g., yelling at the person or withholding some customary benefit such as affection).

And there were even more surprising results from Averill's study. Despite the generally negative connotation of anger, Averill's respondents reported that their anger episodes typically resulted in *constructive* outcomes. Further, both angered individuals and individuals who were the target of someone else's anger agreed that these anger episodes had positive long-term consequences. For example, many respondents indicated that although the feeling of anger was uncomfortable, the final result was a new mutual understanding or a positive change in behavior. Ironically, the potential benefits of anger have received little attention in the research literature. Over the past 50 years, psychologists have generated a rich and extensive body of research on the dark side of anger—human aggression. But far less is known about the more adaptive or constructive functions of anger. It seems that, like most emotions, anger has rich positive as well as negative potential in our social world.

Development of the Anger Response Inventories

In our next line of studies, we attempted to take a much more in-depth look at how individual differences in shame-proneness and guilt-proneness are related to the ways in which people characteristically manage anger across the lifespan. That is, once shame-prone and guilt-prone people become angry, what do they do?

To answer this question, it was necessary to grapple with a new set of measurement issues—this time centering on the assessment of anger-related dimensions. While there are many measures of anger arousal and quite a number of measures of behavioral aggression, psychologists had not developed a measure that assessed the broad range of possible responses to anger. Thus, our first task was to develop a series of parallel child, adolescent, and adult measures that would encompass the full array of cognitive and behavioral responses that people might select when faced with an anger-eliciting event.

The resulting three Anger Response Inventories (ARI for adults— Tangney, Wagner, Marschall, & Gramzow, 1991; ARI-Adol for adolescents—Tangney, Wagner, Gavlas, & Gramzow, 1991; and ARI-C for children—Tangney, Wagner, Hansbarger, & Gramzow, 1991) consist of a series of developmentally appropriate situations that are likely to elicit anger in everyday contexts. As with the SCAAI and TOSCA measures, respondents are asked to imagine themselves in each situation and then rate a number of associated responses.

The ARI scales (see Table 6.1) represent four broad categories of anger-related dimensions: (1) *anger arousal*; (2) *intentions* (e.g., malevolent, constructive); (3) *cognitive and behavioral responses* to anger (including maladaptive behaviors such as aggression, adaptive behaviors such as nonhostile discussion, escapist/diffusing responses, and cognitive reappraisals); and (4) participants' assessment of the likely *long-term consequences* of the anger episode.

Beyond a simple assessment of anger, it is important to assess the *intentions* of an angered individual because the intentions, in part, guide the selection of behavioral responses from a range of alternatives. These intentions are varied and range from clearly constructive to clearly nonconstructive. Averill (1982), for example, identified three factor-analytically derived classes of motives related to anger: Malevolent, Constructive, and Fractious. *Malevolent* motives include expressing dislike, breaking off a relationship, and gaining revenge. *Constructive* motives include strengthening a relationship, asserting authority or independence, bringing about a change for the instigator's own good, and getting the instigator to do something for oneself. *Fractious* motives (i.e., a desire to let off steam) were less varied but emerged as a separate factor.

Behavioral responses to anger are obviously important, as they typically have a direct impact on others. Averill's (1982) extensive historical review of the literature identified a range of aggressive and non-aggressive responses to anger which we have incorporated into the framework for our ARIs. Aggression, for example, can be expressed in a variety of ways. *Direct aggression* involves actions aimed directly at the target of one's anger. Our measures distinguish among physical, verbal, and symbolic forms of direct aggression. *Indirect aggression* involves a more roundabout means of harming the target of one's anger. Our mea-

TABLE 6.1. Assessment of Anger-Related Processes

I. *Anger arousal*

II. *Intentions*
   A. Constructive (desire to fix the situation)
   B. Malevolent (desire to hurt or get back at target)
   C. Fractious (desire to "let off steam") (adults and adolescents only)

III. *Behavioral and cognitive responses to anger*
   A. Maladaptive responses
      1. Direct aggression toward the target
         a. Physical aggression directed at the target (e.g., hitting, shoving, throwing things at the target)
         b. Verbal aggression directed at the target (e.g., yelling, scolding, making a nasty remark)
         c. Symbolic aggression directed at the target (e.g., shaking a fist, slamming a door in the target's face)
      2. Indirect aggression
         a. Malediction—bad-mouthing the target to a third party
         b. Harm—harming something important to the target or denying a customary benefit (e.g., destroying property of target, refusing to speak to the target)
      3. Displaced aggression (against someone or something not directly involved)
         a. Physical aggression against another person
         b. Verbal aggression against another person
         c. Aggression toward a nonhuman object (not connected to the target) (e.g., kicking the dog, hitting a wall)
      4. Self-directed aggression (e.g., berating one's self for the situation)
      5. Anger held in (brooding, ruminating over the incident without expressing)

   B. Adaptive behaviors
      1. Nonhostile discussion with target of anger
      2. Direct corrective action

   C. Escapist/diffusing responses
      1. Attempts to diffuse anger (e.g., distracting activities)
      2. Minimizing importance of incident
      3. Removal (leaving situation)
      4. Doing nothing

   D. Cognitive reappraisals
      1. Reinterpreting the motives or actions of the target (e.g., "He didn't mean it," "She was just trying to help")
      2. Reinterpreting one's own role in the situation (e.g., "It was partly my fault; maybe I should have been more careful")

IV. *Long-term consequences*
   A. For the self
   B. For the target
   C. For the relationship

Note. Adapted from Tangney, Barlow, et al. (1996). Copyright 1996 by the American Psychological Association. Adapted by permission.

sures distinguished between two different forms of *indirect aggression*: withholding or harming something important to the instigator, and *malediction* (talking badly behind the instigator's back to get revenge). *Displaced aggression* involves aggressive acts "displaced" onto someone or something unrelated to the target of one's anger. The ARI measures assess three types of *displaced aggression*: physical and verbal aggression directed toward uninvolved people, and aggression directed toward nonhuman objects.

In addition to other-directed aggressive responses to anger, anger can also result in negative behavior directed toward the self. Two types of "self-oriented" responses were included under the heading of maladaptive responses to anger. The *Self-Directed Aggression* scale assesses a tendency to berate oneself or to become disproportionately angry with oneself for the anger eliciting event. The *Anger Held In* scale, similar to that of Spielberger et al. (1985), assesses a tendency to ruminate over the event without expressing one's anger directly.

The ARIs are unique not only in their comprehensive assessment of various forms of aggression; indeed, perhaps the most novel aspect of the ARIs is their consideration of *nonaggressive responses* to anger. We distinguished among three broad classes of nonaggressive anger-management strategies: *adaptive behaviors, escapist/diffusing responses*, and *cognitive reappraisals*. Two types of clearly adaptive behaviors were identified in Averill's (1982) studies: rational, nonhostile *discussion with the target* of one's anger, and direct *corrective action* aimed at "fixing" some key aspect of the anger-eliciting situation (e.g., changing lanes to remedy being tailgated). The second cluster of nonaggressive responses—escapist/diffusing responses—are not clearly adaptive or maladaptive. These include attempts to *diffuse* the anger (e.g., by engaging in some distracting activity), efforts to *minimize* the importance of the event (e.g., "Oh well, it wasn't that big of a deal anyway"), *removal* (e.g., walking away, leaving the situation), and simply *doing nothing*. We also considered people's tendency to subsequently engage in cognitive reappraisals of the anger-inducing incident (e.g., reinterpreting the instigator's motives). Such reappraisals may occur in lieu of behavioral responses and may lead to a significant reduction in anger arousal and malevolent intentions, to the extent that they alter attributions regarding the target's responsibility for or controllability of the event (Berkowitz, 1993; C. A. Smith & Ellsworth, 1985). In fact, such reappraisals were often associated with positive outcomes in Averill's (1982) studies. The ARIs assess two types of cognitive reappraisals: reappraisals of the target's role include reconsidering the other person's intentions, motives, or actual behaviors in bringing about the anger-eliciting event (e.g., "Well, maybe he didn't really mean to do it," "Maybe she couldn't help it"); reappraisals of the self's role include reassessments of the participant's own intentions, motives, or behaviors that may have contributed to the anger-eliciting event (e.g., "I wonder if *I* made a mistake").

Finally, participants are asked to estimate the likely long-term consequences of anger-eliciting episodes, considering the event itself and their anger-related responses. The ARIs assess the likely consequences for the self, consequences for the target of the anger, and consequences for the relationship between the participant and the target.

Empirical Links to Shame and Guilt

Since developing the ARIs, we have administered these measures to several thousand children, adolescents, and adults. One thing that's clear is that people vary a great deal in how they manage and express feelings of anger. Some people are inclined to aggress. In their fury, they lash out at those around them and take steps to "even the score." Others tend to hold their anger in. They stew over perceived injustices without directly expressing their ire. Or they attempt to ignore, minimize, or distract themselves from their anger. Still others orient themselves in a constructive direction. They draw on their anger to make changes for the better—opening lines of communication, resolving conflict, and setting things right. What accounts for these individual differences in anger management strategies? What factors "tip the balance," allowing people to make constructive—as opposed to destructive—use of their anger?

To address these questions, we focused on individual differences in moral-emotional style (shame-proneness and guilt-proneness), in a cross-sectional developmental study of 302 children (grades 4–6), 427 adolescents (grades 7–11), 176 college students, and 194 adult travelers passing through a large urban airport (Tangney, Wagner, et al., 1996). Participants in each subsample completed the age-appropriate versions of the ARI and TOSCA measures.

Across all ages, proneness to shame was substantially correlated with anger arousal, thus replicating our earlier findings with more traditional measures of anger. Perhaps more importantly, across individuals of all ages (from 8 years of age through adulthood), shame-prone individuals are not only more prone to anger, in general, but they are also more likely to do unconstructive things with their anger, compared to their less-shame-prone peers. Shame-proneness was related to malevo-lent and fractious (e.g., a desire to "let off steam") intentions, as well as a likelihood of engaging in direct physical, verbal, and symbolic aggres-sion, indirect aggression (e.g., harming something important to the tar-get, talking behind the target's back), all kinds of displaced aggression, self-directed aggression, and anger held in (a ruminative unexpressed anger). In contrast, shame-prone individuals were not particularly in-clined to discuss the matter with the target of their anger in a nonhostile, constructive fashion. Rather, they were more likely simply to walk away from the situation, compared to their non-shame-prone peers. Finally, shame-proneness was associated with negative long-term consequences as a result of the entire episode of anger.

The findings regarding proneness to guilt were another story entirely. Guilt-proneness was generally associated with constructive means of handling anger. Proneness to "shame-free" guilt was positively correlated with constructive intentions and negatively correlated with all indices of direct, indirect, and displaced aggression. Instead, com-pared to their non-guilt-prone peers, guilt-prone individuals were much more likely to report that they would engage in constructive behavior such as nonhostile discussion with the target of their anger and direct corrective action. Guilt-proneness was also associated with reported at-tempts to diffuse the feeling of anger (e.g., by engaging in some distract-ing activity) and with cognitive reappraisals of the target's role in the sit-uation (e.g., "Maybe he didn't mean to do it") and of the self's role in the situation (e.g., "Maybe I had something to do with the situation"). Finally, proneness to shame-free guilt was associated with respondents' assessments of positive long-term consequences as a result of the entire episode of anger.[1]

The relationship of shame and guilt to these anger-related dimen-sions appears to be quite robust. The findings are largely independent of the influence of social desirability. Moreover, these results were subse-quently replicated in a study of 256 college students (Tangney, 1995b) and 216 romantically involved couples (Tangney, 1995c).

In sum, results across diverse samples and studies indicate that shame-prone individuals of all ages (from early childhood through late adulthood) experience more anger than their less-shame-prone peers. Moreover, once angered, the shame-prone person's subsequent motiva-tions and behaviors differ considerably from those who are less shame-prone. How do we understand these results?

SHAMED INTO ANGER OR WITHDRAWAL?:
GUILT-TRIPPED INTO CONSTRUCTIVE CHANGE?

Earlier, we suggested that the shame-prone person's anger often represents a defensive, retaliative reaction to shame. Thus, it is not surprising
to find that shame-proneness is associated with malevolent and fractious intentions, and a likelihood of engaging in all manner of direct, indirect, and displaced aggression. Consider, for example, a shame-prone
midlevel office manager who makes an obvious mistake and is suddenly
faced with a very public failure. Feeling shamed, humiliated, and angry,
he may lash out at his subordinates (in person and in their evaluations),
irrationally placing the blame on their shoulders. At the next opportunity by the watercooler, he may viciously malign his boss to a colleague,
insinuating that his difficulties stem from poor upper management. At
the extreme, he might even engage in some covert acts of sabotage toward the company. Each of these aggressive responses may serve to
lessen his painful feelings of shame.

Alternatively, shamed individuals may choose to withdraw from
shame- and anger-eliciting situations. Individual differences in proneness to shame were not only related to active aggressive responses but
also to a passive, internalized strategy for managing situations involving
interpersonal conflict. Shame-proneness was clearly associated with anger held in (a ruminative, unexpressed anger), self-directed hostility,
and a tendency to withdraw from anger-related situations. For example,
the humiliated shame-prone manager may opt to repress his rage and
instead engage in ruminative anger at the self and everyone involved.
Following the day of humiliation, he may call in sick or simply withdraw from colleagues by hunkering down in his office behind a closed
door.

In short, when faced with situations involving interpersonal conflict, shame-prone people appear to adopt one of two strategies when
faced with situations involving interpersonal conflict—active aggression or passive withdrawal—neither of which is likely to result in a
favorable outcome for the situation or relationship at hand. Not surprisingly, shame-prone individuals in our studies reported that the likely
long-term consequences of the everyday episodes of anger would be
pretty grim.

In contrast, guilt-prone individuals appear to adopt a third, more
proactive and constructive strategy for managing everyday anger. Con-

sistent with Baumeister et al.'s (1994) observation that guilt serves a range of relationship-enhancing functions, proneness to "shame-free" guilt was positively correlated with constructive strategies for managing anger and conflict. For example, a guilt-prone midlevel manager may initially feel some anger and resentment at being publicly called on the carpet for his oversight. However, feeling guilt rather than shame, he has less call to become defensive. Reviewing the situation, he may more readily accept responsibility for the failure, or at least be more inclined to explain the circumstances leading up to the problem. Feeling resentment toward his boss for the public castigation, he is apt to tactfully but directly suggest that future issues be handled one-on-one. And, perhaps most importantly, he is inclined to get down to the business of figuring out how to avoid similar problems in the future.

What allows guilt-prone individuals to make constructive use of their anger? First, guilt-prone individuals are apt to *construe* anger-eliciting situations differently than shame-prone individuals. Because guilt involves a negative evaluation of a specific behavior, somewhat apart from the global self, guilt experiences are less likely to involve severe threats to the self and hence are less likely to invoke a defensive, retaliative sort of anger. In short, guilt-prone individuals are not typically saddled with irrational shame-based anger aroused in a desperate attempt to rescue a devalued self. Rather, their anger is more likely to focus on reality-based violations and infractions committed by themselves or others. At issue, then, is a real and concrete infraction which can be addressed in a direct and rational manner with the perpetrator or which can be "fixed" by some other direct constructive action. Such strategies are not readily available to shame-prone individuals when they become irrationally angry as a means of extricating themselves from painful feelings of shame. Second, guilt-prone individuals are less likely to be impaired by global and debilitating feelings of shame, and thus may feel more *able* to take direct, constructive action when faced with situations involving interpersonal conflict. These guilt-prone people's sense of self-efficacy is unimpaired by the experience of shame. Moreover, several studies suggest that guilt-prone individuals have better interpersonal skills, compared to their less-guilt-prone peers (Tangney, 1994; Tangney, Wagner, Burggraf, et al., 1991). Thus, guilt-prone individuals may be especially well placed to make use of a key adaptive response to anger—rational, nonhostile discussion with the target of their anger. Given their enhanced sense of self-efficacy and relatively strong interpersonal skills, guilt-prone individuals may be more inclined to "talk things out" with others who have angered them, in part because they view this strategy as likely to result in a successful outcome. Third and finally, guilt-prone individuals' enhanced capacity for empathy (Tangney, 1991, 1994; Tangney, Wagner, Burggraf, et al., 1991) undoubtedly shapes their responses to anger. Such feelings of other-oriented empathy no doubt contribute to the guilt-prone person's tendency to reappraise the target's role and intentions in anger-eliciting situations. And this ability to take the other person's perspective, even when angered, likely paves the way to constructive intentions and actions (such as a nonhostile discussion with the target of the anger) while diffusing malevolent intentions and aggressive behaviors aimed at harming or "getting back" at the target.

FEELINGS OF SHAME AND ANGER "IN THE MOMENT"

So far, we have been considering the implications of shame-prone and guilt-prone dispositions or traits. How do individual differences in the tendency to experience shame (or guilt) across a range of situations relate to people's strategies for managing anger? In interpreting these results, we have speculated about the effects of situation-specific feelings of shame on, for example, the ability to empathize, the likelihood of becoming angry, and subsequent means of managing that anger.

But so far the data have been at the trait or dispositional level. And as researchers have long noted, these sorts of correlational data at the level of dispositions are open to all sorts of alternative explanations. For example, it is possible (although unlikely, in our view) that shame-prone people experience a lot of shame in some situations and a lot of anger in other situations, but rarely both in the same event. Under such circumstances, one would still observe a substantial correlation between dispositional shame and dispositional anger—the same as if shame-prone people's episodes of shame in turn provoked defensive anger reactions across many situations. Much of our speculation about the *dynamics* between shame, guilt, and anger has been just that—speculation, as we try to understand the meaning of relationships among dispositional measures.

Relatively little research has explicitly examined shame and anger in specific situations, but two earlier studies are suggestive of a functional link between these two emotions. In a study of undergraduates, Wicker et al. (1983) found that participants were more likely to report a desire to punish *others*, as well as a desire to hide, when rating personal shame versus guilt experiences. Tangney, Miller, et al. (1996), too, found a similar trend among college students who reported more feelings of anger in connection with narrative accounts of shame versus guilt experiences.

More recently, we have greatly expanded our research concerning feelings of shame in specific situations. We have been looking at the implications of situation-specific feelings of shame and guilt in two independent studies: one study of about 200 romantically involved couples, and a parallel study of about 100 adolescents and their parents. The focus of these studies was on specific real-life episodes of anger. Our aim was to identify factors (situational and dispositional) that foster constructive as opposed to destructive responses to anger in everyday contexts. To this end, we conducted in-depth interviews with couples and families concerning recent episodes of shared anger. For example, in our couples' study (Tangney, Barlow, Borenstein, & Marschall, 2001), initially the couple worked together to identify (but not discuss) two recent events involving anger—one in which the boyfriend had angered the girlfriend, and one in which the girlfriend had angered the boyfriend. Partners were then interviewed separately about their perceptions, thoughts, and behaviors during the event.

Many types of anger-eliciting events were identified by the couples. The events varied along numerous dimensions, but one factor we were particularly interested in was whether the event (the offense) elicited feelings of shame in the victim. Victims were asked if the event had involved "a loss of pride, self-esteem or personal worth." (We provided this colloquial description of situation-specific shame, having found that people tend to defend against the word "shame" itself. As discussed in Chapter 4, feelings of shame are conceptually akin to sudden, transient losses of "state" self-esteem—see Figure 4.1.) Thus, there were two types of anger events—one in which the victim was shamed *and* angry, and the other in which the victim was angered but not shamed.

Results from our first set of analyses strongly supported the hypothesized link between shame and maladaptive responses to anger. First, victims of the shame-related anger events experienced more anger than did victims in the non-shame-related events. Second, shamed victims were more likely to report malevolent and fractious intentions. That is, they tended to be oriented toward getting back at their partner and letting off steam, rather than trying to fix the situation. Third, shamed victims responded to their anger differently from nonshamed victims—they behaved differently. Here, we observed some interesting sex differences. Shamed boyfriends showed a tendency to respond with a range of direct and indirect forms of aggression—behaviors intended to cause harm in one way or another to the perpetrating girlfriend. These shamed boyfriends also were prone to a ruminative anger held in (thinking about the situation over and over, becoming more and more angry). Whereas shamed boyfriends showed a tendency to lash out at their girlfriends, shamed girlfriends showed a tendency to engage in displaced aggression (aggression displaced onto people and things other than the boyfriend), as well as self-directed hostility. Fourth, not surprisingly, shamed victims did not feel very good about the way they handled their anger. Shamed girlfriends reported that they felt more embarrassed, anxious, sad, shamed, and surprised about how they handled their anger. (There was also a trend for shamed girlfriends to feel proud—perhaps because of the restraint many showed in these situations.) The aggressive shamed boyfriends reported that they felt dominant, sad, and ashamed about how they handled their anger. Fifth, these apparently maladaptive expressions of anger did not result in any positive behavior on the part of the shame-inducing perpetrators (especially according to the victims' accounts). Perpetrator's responses to the aggressive retaliation of shamed victims centered on anger, resentment, defiance, and denial—rather than, for example, apologies and attempts to fix the situation. Finally, we asked the couples about the long-term consequences of the entire anger episode—considering the event itself, the victim's responses, and the perpetrator's reactions. In no case did the shame-related anger episodes result in more beneficial consequences than the non-shame-related episodes. The consensus was that the situations involving shamed boyfriends were the most destructive, particularly from the girlfriends' perspective. (This makes a great deal of sense, considering the shamed boyfriends' tendency toward overt aggression.) The couples identified the situations involving shamed girlfriends as less problematic. (This is where the girlfriends were prone to engage in displaced and self-directed aggression.) Here, there was a trend for the girlfriends themselves to note negative long-term consequences for the relationship. Boyfriends were, not surprisingly, oblivious.

In sum, these findings regarding situation-specific feelings of shame in the midst of couples' real-life episodes of anger converge nicely with the results from the dispositional studies linking trait shame with trait anger and characteristic maladaptive responses to anger. And, as discussed in greater detail in Chapter 10, these data provide a powerful empirical example of the shame-rage spiral described by H. B. Lewis (1971) and Scheff (1987).

SUMMARY AND CONCLUSIONS

In this chapter, we have discussed some of the different ways that people react to feelings of shame and guilt, focusing particularly on anger and aggression. When people feel shame over a particular failure or transgression, the shame reflects on who they are as a person. Consequently, it is extremely difficult to fix the problem—because the problem lies with the self. Because reparative action doesn't get to the core of the problem, shame-prone people often attempt to deflect nasty feelings of shame. One option is to withdraw, escaping the shame-inducing situation. Another common strategy involves shifting the blame to others. Blaming *others* (instead of the self) can help people defend and preserve their self-esteem while also regaining some sense of agency and control. Feeling anger, the self is "reactivated." Although defensive anger may help in the short term, reducing immediate feelings of shame, the long-term effects on interpersonal relationships are likely to be bleak. This is especially the case because, once angered, shame-prone people manage and express their anger in an aggressive and destructive manner.

In contrast, because feelings of guilt are typically less painful and less ego threatening, guilt is less likely to provoke defensive anger, denial, and aggression. Rather, guilt appears to facilitate feelings of other-oriented empathy (see Chapter 5), curbing anger, and encouraging more constructive means of communicating anger and dissatisfaction. Consistent with Baumeister et al.'s (1994) observation that guilt serves a range of relationship-enhancing functions, proneness to "shame-free" guilt has been positively correlated with constructive strategies for managing anger and conflict.

This chapter has described one of the great surprises from our program of research on shame and guilt. Contrary to folk wisdom, feelings of shame actually provoke other-directed anger, rather than inhibiting anger and aggression. These findings were a reminder to us of why it is so important to collect data—because our assumptions about how people behave are not always on the mark.

NOTE

1. One cluster of scales—the Escapist/Diffusing Responses—showed some interesting developmental trends. Among children and adolescents, these dimensions were consistently positively correlated with guilt and, with the exception of Removal, largely unrelated to shame. Among older participants, however, the shame and guilt correlates were much less clear cut. This pattern of findings is consistent with some of our other findings which showed a developmental shift in the long-term consequences of these Escapist/Diffusing Responses. For children, such attempts to escape or diffuse the anger-eliciting situation appear to have fairly positive outcomes. In other words, it appears that anything children can do to "keep a lid" on their anger is an adaptive strategy. Such efforts at anger suppression seem to become less adaptive with age. Among college students and adults, direct constructive responses (e.g., corrective action and attempts to discuss the matter with the target of the anger) were most strongly linked to positive long-term consequences.

Chapter 7

SHAME, GUILT,
AND PSYCHOPATHOLOGY

In the last few chapters, we have described the many dark sides of shame. Research consistently links shame to poor interpersonal skills, an impaired capacity for empathy, feelings of anger and hostility, and maladaptive strategies for managing anger. On this there is little controversy. But what about guilt? Over the years, guilt has had a pretty bad reputation, too. No one wants a "guilt-inducing" mother. Almost as bad is a "guilt-tripping" friend. Countless jokes have been made about the curse of Jewish or Catholic guilt. According to numerous self-help books, guilt is something one can best do without. And therapists, too, often regard guilt as a problem to be "worked through."

In light of these common assumptions, the reader might be surprised by the picture of guilt that has emerged in the research so far. Guilt has been consistently linked to social competence not incompetence, to an enhanced capacity for other-oriented empathy, and to constructive strategies for managing anger. But what about a person's own level of psychological adjustment? Does the tendency to experience guilt over one's transgressions, to feel empathy for one's victims, and to set aside one's own needs and desires in favor of the needs of others ultimately lead to increases in anxiety and depression? Indeed, does guilt serve adaptive functions at the interpersonal and societal level only at considerable cost to the psychological well-being of the individual?

There is some debate on this point in the current literature. Before we present what the research has shown, we first take a historical look at the role of shame and guilt in theories of psychopathology. Psychologists working from a range of theoretical perspectives have speculated about the implications of shame and guilt for the formation of psychological symptoms. But after more than a century of contemplation and speculation, there is still no clear consensus on the degree to which guilt is maladaptive. As it turns out, the answer depends in part on how one defines shame and guilt, and to a larger extent on how one assesses these emotion styles (see Harder, 1995; Tangney et al., 1995). A careful examination of the empirical literature shows that when measures are used that are sensitive to H. B. Lewis's (1971) self versus behavior distinction (e.g., scenario-based methods assessing shame-proneness and guilt-proneness with respect to specific situations), guilt doesn't look so bad after all. Nonetheless, an intriguing question remains: Is there such a thing as "maladaptive" guilt? Researchers in this area continue to engage in lively discussion and debate on this clinically important issue.

THE ROLE OF SHAME AND GUILT
IN PSYCHOPATHOLOGY: A CENTURY OF THEORY

Early Psychoanalytic Perspectives

Historically, guilt—not shame—has been identified as the culprit in a host of psychological disorders. Interestingly, in his early writings, Freud (1896/1953a) considered the potential relevance of both shame and guilt to psychological disorders. In 1905, he discussed shame as a reaction formation against sexually exhibitionistic impulses, but in his later writings he pretty much abandoned the notion of shame, focusing instead on a more cognitive conceptualization of the sense of guilt arising from ego/superego conflicts.

From Freud's (1923/1961d) perspective, a sense of guilt comes about when forbidden wishes or deeds clash with the moral standards of the ever-vigilant superego. In turn, the superego retaliates in a manner that often leads to psychological symptoms. The superego, and its guilt and anxiety-inducing tactics, can be traced back to the resolution of the Oedipal conflict. Freud's (1905/1953b, 1914/1957, 1923/1961d, 1924/1961c, 1925/1961b) accounts of the dynamics of the Oedipal drama are exceedingly complex, spanning several decades of development and revision. But, in a nutshell, children experience sexual, possessive feelings for the mother during the Oedipal period that provoke feelings of rivalry, jealousy, and hostility toward the father. The child (most clearly the male child) has fantasies of doing away with the father so that he can take the father's place as mother's partner. But these fantasies inevitably raise the specter of disastrous consequences. The arch-rival (father) looms as an omnipotent, threatening figure. He becomes larger than life as the child projects his own jealousy and hostility onto this all-powerful rival parent. As a result, the child comes to fear severe retaliation—eventually the ultimate retaliation: castration. Fear of cas-tration is intensified when, at about the same age, the young child dis-covers that some children (little girls) already lack the prized penis; moreover, such fear may be exacerbated by implicit or explicit threats of castration for early masturbatory activity. In any event, as the child's sexual attachment to the mother heightens, the child's fear of retaliatory castration becomes even more ingrained. In a desperate attempt to cope with this terrifying dilemma, the child ultimately engages in a "super-repression" of sexual impulses, toward the mother and in general. This massive repression is bolstered and reinforced by corresponding intense identification with the father. And this highly charged father identifica-tion forms the foundation of the superego, which continues to develop as the child is exposed to a range of socialization experiences.[1] In essence, then, mature guilt has its roots in earlier Oedipal castration anxiety. Fear of castration by the father for rather specific sexual and ag-gressive impulses vis-à-vis the parents is transformed into more general feelings of guilt and anxiety for all manner of transgressions. In the post-Oedipal years, guilt and anxiety are generated not by the father, per se, but by the internalized authority of the superego.

From Freud's perspective, problematic guilt "complexes" and asso-ciated psychological symptoms (e.g., anxiety, depression, somatization) are essentially due to a superego "gone awry." More specifically, the root of many forms of psychopathology can be traced to excessive guilt stemming from some perturbation in the Oedipal phase of develop-ment: constitutionally based excessive libidinal urges, an overpunitive father, a seductive mother, chance mishaps during early masturbatory exploration, and so forth.

Freud was much less systematic in his treatment of shame. Re-cently, a number of theorists have suggested that Freud's relative neglect of shame may have been due to his focus on a conflict-defense model of psychological functioning and to his failure to distinguish between ego and self (H. B. Lewis, 1987a; S. B. Miller, 1985; A. P. Morrison, 1989;

Tangney, 1994). A. P. Morrison (1989), for example, suggested that Freud might have further elaborated on the nature and implications of shame had he pursued the concepts of ego-ideal, narcissism, and self-regard (so central to shame) in greater depth. Instead, Freud's work subsequent to 1914 focused to a much greater extent on guilt-inducing Oedipal issues and on a structural theory that emphasized intrapsychic conflict among ego, id, and superego (with little regard for the more self-relevant ego-ideal).

H. B. Lewis (1971) has suggested that in developing a theory that focused almost exclusively on guilt Freud may have mislabeled his patients' shame experiences as guilt experiences. As discussed in Chapter 2, a key difference between these two emotions centers on negative evaluations of a specific behavior versus the global self. As noted above, a number of contemporary theorists (H. B. Lewis, 1987a; S. B. Miller, 1985; A. P. Morrison, 1989) have pointed out that Freud's framework was ill equipped to accommodate this distinction because he did not distinguish a concept of self as distinct from the ego in his structural model. From a classical Freudian perspective, then, both self-directed evaluations and behavior-directed evaluations are equally "ego" relevant—with both being labeled as "guilt."

An Emerging Recognition of Shame

In subsequent years, a number of psychoanalytically oriented theorists made explicit attempts to distinguish between shame and guilt (e.g., Hartmann & Loewenstein, 1962; Jacobson, 1954; Piers & Singer, 1953). Freud's (1914/1957) previously abandoned notion of an ego-ideal was later picked up by ego psychologists, who elaborated on the distinction between ego-ideal and superego (or conscience) proper. In an attempt to apply this distinction to a conceptualization of shame and guilt, Piers and Singer (1953) defined guilt as a reaction to clashes between the ego and superego, and shame as a reaction to clashes between the ego and the ego-ideal. Transgressions in conflict with superego prohibitions were thought to lead to feelings of guilt and anxiety with its roots in fears of castration (similar to Freud's own notions), whereas failure to measure up to the ego-ideal was thought to lead to feelings of shame and inferiority, and consequent fears of loss of love and abandonment. This neo-Freudian distinction between shame and guilt can be seen as a precursor to H. B. Lewis's (1971) later distinction between self and behavior concerns, and it is consistent with Erikson's (1950) descriptions of shame as global exposed self-doubt versus guilt over mis-guided behavior (initiative).

The neo-Freudian structural distinction is not without its prob-lems. For example, Hartmann and Loewenstein (1962) voiced concerns about the practical utility of such a structural distinction. And more re-cently, Lindsay-Hartz (1984) provided compelling contradictory evi-dence from an in-depth study of the phenomenology of shame and guilt. Her results strongly suggest that shame typically results from the recognition that "we are who we do not want to be" (Lindsay-Hartz, 1984, p. 697)—a *negative* ideal—rather than from a recognition that we have failed to live up to some *positive* ideal.

In recent years, shame has gained a much more prominent role in psychodynamic theory. With the development of self psychology, psychoanalytically oriented clinicians and theorists have embraced the self-relevant shame experience as a key component of a range of psy-chological disorders (Goldberg, 1991; Kohut, 1971; Lansky, 1987; A. P. Morrison, 1989; N. K. Morrison, 1987; Nathanson, 1987b, 1987c). These theories vary in the functional role assigned to shame: in some, shame is viewed as the cause of psychopathology; in others, it is viewed as the result of a fundamental defect in the self system. These theories, however, share a common focus on shame and, somewhat ironically, a corresponding de-emphasis of guilt. In fact, in some cases, the construct of guilt, as distinct from shame, is largely neglected and so, again, as in traditional Freudian theory, the distinction between these two emotions is lost.

The recent surge of interest in shame extends beyond the psycho-analytic literature. Shame has been cited as a significant factor in family-systems-oriented conceptualizations of substance abuse, depression, eating disorders, and child abuse (Fossum & Mason, 1986), in the codependency literature (Bradshaw, 1988; Potter-Efron, 1989), and in social-cognitive conceptualizations of eating disorders (Rodin et al., 1985).

CONTEMPORARY COGNITIVE PERSPECTIVES

The recent focus on the pathogenic implications of shame makes good sense from a cognitive theoretical perspective as well. For example, H. B. Lewis noted parallels between her conceptualization of shame and guilt and attributional patterns frequently discussed in connection with depression (e.g., Abramson et al., 1978; Beck, 1983). Although the attributional literature makes few explicit references to shame and guilt, these emotions involve both affective and cognitive components. What's more, the cognitive aspects of shame and guilt can be readily understood in attributional terms (Hoblitzelle, 1987a, 1987b; H. B. Lewis, 1987c). Shame—in its focus on the entire self—can be construed as an affective state stemming from internal, stable, and global attributions. Guilt—in its focus on specific behaviors—can be construed as an affective state arising from internal, specific, and presumably less stable attributions. Thus, when the cognitive components of these affective states are considered, the distinction between guilt and shame bears some resemblance to Janoff-Bulman's (1979) distinction between behavioral and characterological self-blame.[2] To the extent that characterological self-blame (the tendency to make internal, global, and stable attributions for negative events) has been theoretically and empirically linked to depression (for a review, see Robins, 1988), the attributional literature is consistent with the notion that there may be a special link between depression and proneness to shame but not proneness to guilt.

It should be noted that because many theorists neglect the distinction between shame and guilt, the term "guilt" is often used to describe the villain in the formation of psychological symptoms. For example, the DSM-IV (American Psychiatric Association, 1994) cites "feelings of worthlessness or excessive or inappropriate guilt" as a symptom of major depressive episodes (p. 327), but the manual is unclear whether feelings of worthlessness (akin to shame) and guilt are seen as essentially synonymous. The widely used Beck Depression Inventory (BDI) contains an item about frequency of guilt experiences (e.g., "I feel quite guilty most of the time"). Similarly, in his description of introjective depression, Blatt (1974) discussed the role of guilt at length. But a closer reading of the phenomenology of introjective depression suggests that shame, not guilt, may be central to this type of depression. Blatt (1974) stated that introjective depression involves "feelings of being unworthy, unlovable . . . of having failed to live up to expectations, . . . a constant self-scrutiny and evaluation . . . and extensive demands for perfection" (p. 117). In this, Blatt has vividly described the key elements of shame.

In sum, cognitive theories—although not addressing shame and guilt per se—suggest that shame is likely to be the more "pathogenic" emotion, particularly in connection with depression. Feelings of "shame-free" guilt, on the other hand, look fairly functional from a cognitive perspective. When people make internal but specific and unstable attributions for their wrongdoings, possibilities for change or repair are likely to be readily apparent. Compared to feelings of shame, those of guilt are less likely to cause an individual to become mired in a sense of hopeless self-blame.

IS GUILT ADAPTIVE OR MALADAPTIVE?: THE CONTROVERSY CONTINUES

This is not to say that among current theorists there is clear consensus concerning the benign nature of guilt. Harder (1995; Harder et al., 1992; Harder & Lewis, 1987), has strongly asserted that tendencies to experience both shame and guilt should be related to psychological symptoms, citing H. B. Lewis's (1971) conceptualization of the *differential* roles of shame and guilt in psychopathology.

Drawing on her earlier work with Witkin and colleagues (1954; also Witkin, Lewis, & Weil, 1968), H. B. Lewis (1971) hypothesized that individual differences in cognitive style (i.e., field dependence vs. field independence) lead to contrasting modes of superego functioning (i.e., shame-proneness and guilt-proneness), and together these cognitive and affective styles lead people down divergent paths of symptom formation. She suggested that the global, less differentiated self of the field-dependent individual is vulnerable to the global, less differentiated experience of shame—and ultimately to affective disorders (particularly depression). In contrast, the more clearly differentiated self of the field-independent individual is vulnerable to the experience of guilt (which requires a differentiation between self and behavior), and also to obsessive and paranoid symptoms involving vigilance of the "field," separate from the self.

This is one point where our thinking diverges substantially from that of Lewis (1971). We believe there are compelling reasons to expect that psychological symptoms would be associated with a predisposition to shame but *not* guilt. Once the critical distinction is made between shame and guilt, guilt doesn't look so bad. Moving beyond the everyday understanding of guilt as self-directed bad feelings—instead viewing guilt as a sense of remorse or regret in connection with some *specific behavior* rather than as a global condemnation of the self—one might argue that, if anything, guilt should be *adaptive*. In guilt, there is an implicit distinction between self and behavior that essentially protects the self from unwarranted global devaluation while keeping the door open for changing the guilt-inducing behavior and/or for making amends for its consequences. From this perspective, guilt is a hopeful, future-oriented moral-emotional experience. Thus, a tendency toward "shame-free" guilt should be unrelated to psychological symptoms.

EMPIRICAL STUDIES OF SHAME
AND GUILT IN PSYCHOPATHOLOGY

What do the data show? Well, it depends. It depends to a great extent on the type of measure used to assess guilt. Studies employing adjective checklist-type (and other globally worded) measures of shame and guilt have found that both shame-prone and guilt-prone styles are associated with psychological symptoms (Friedman, 1999; Harder, 1995; Harder et al., 1992; Harder & Lewis, 1987; Jones & Kugler, 1993; Meehan et al., 1996; O'Connor, Berry, & Weiss, 1999). These studies did not show consistent differences in the types of symptoms associated with shame versus guilt, as H. B. Lewis (1971) had suggested. But clearly, in these studies, guilt emerges as problematic.

On the other hand, a very different pattern of results emerges when measures are used that are sensitive to Lewis's (1971) self versus behavior distinction, such as our TOSCA measures, which assess shame-proneness and guilt-proneness with respect to specific situations. (As discussed in Chapter 3, there are a number of different strategies for measuring guilt—some more theoretically consistent than others.) In numerous independent studies of children and adults, we found that proneness to "shame-free" guilt was largely unrelated to psychological maladjustment, whereas proneness to shame (as expected) was linked to a host of psychological problems (Tangney, 1994; Tangney et al., 1995; Tangney, Wagner, & Gramzow, 1992; Gramzow & Tangney, 1992; Burggraf & Tangney, 1990; Tangney, Wagner, Burggraf, et al., 1991). Other labs, too, using scenario-based methods, report a differential relationship between shame and guilt on the one hand and psychological problems on the other (Chandler-Holtz, 1999; O'Connor et al., 1999; Shaefer, 2000; Shiffler, 1998; but see Ferguson, Stegge, Miller, & Olson, 1999). Similarly, using the DEQ, Darvill, Johnson, and Danko (1992) found that, compared to guilt, shame was more highly associated with neuroticism.

Results from three independent studies of undergraduates illustrate the point nicely and closely replicate those of Tangney, Wagner, and Gramzow (1992). To assess proneness to shame and proneness to guilt, participants in all three studies completed the Test of Self-Conscious Affect (TOSCA; Tangney et al., 1989). To assess psychological symptoms, participants in all the studies completed the Symptom Checklist-90 (SCL-90; Derogatis et al., 1973). The SCL-90 is a widely used clinical rating scale composed of 90 symptoms, and it is appropriate for use with both psychiatric and nonclinical populations. It provides nine clinical subscales: Somatization, Obsessive–Compulsive, Interpersonal Sensitivity (assessing feelings of personal inadequacy or inferiority), Depression, Anxiety, Hostility, Phobic Anxiety, Paranoid Ideation, and Psychoticism. Participants in Studies 1 and 2 also completed the Beck Depression Inventory (BDI).

As expected, the tendency to experience shame across a range of situations was strongly related to psychological maladjustment in general (see Table A.4 in Appendix A for more detail). Despite the restricted range of psychopathology in this largely young and healthy sample, all 12 indices of psychopathology were positively and significantly correlated with shame-proneness. Guilt-proneness, on the other hand, was negligibly related to psychopathology, and proneness to "shame-free" guilt was in some cases *negatively* related to psychological symptoms.[3]

We should emphasize that the results involving shame, shown in Appendix A, Table A.4, are entirely consistent with the results from other labs. In fact, there is no debate regarding the pathogenic nature of shame. Empirical research consistently demonstrates a relationship between proneness to shame and a whole host of psychological symptoms, including depression, anxiety, eating disorder symptoms, subclinical sociopathy, and low self-esteem (Allan, Gilbert, & Goss, 1994; Brodie, 1995; Cook, 1988, 1991; Gramzow & Tangney, 1992; Harder, 1995; Harder et al., 1992; Harder & Lewis, 1987; Hoblitzelle, 1987; Sanftner et al., 1995; Tangney, 1993a, 1993b; Tangney et al., 1995; Tangney, Wagner, Burggraf, et al., 1991; Tangney, Wagner, & Gramzow, 1992). This relationship appears to be robust across a range of measurement methods (the assessment of shame is less "delicate" than guilt, not requiring a consideration of specific behaviors) and across diverse age groups and populations.

IS PRONENESS TO SHAME JUST A REINVENTION OF ATTRIBUTIONAL STYLE?

As discussed in Chapter 4, the cognitive components of shame and guilt can be conceptualized in attributional terms: shame, in its focus on the entire self, involves internal, stable, and global attributions; guilt, in its focus on specific behaviors, involves internal, specific, and presumably unstable attributions. Much research suggests that the tendency to make internal, stable and global, attributions for negative events leads to depression (Robins, 1988). Given the observed links between shame and psychopathology, particularly depression and anxiety, it seems important to determine whether these findings are simply a reflection of participants' attributional style. If so, a consideration of shame may be largely superfluous to our understanding of psychological maladjustment, beyond what current cognitive theories have to offer. Individual differences in cognitive style may provide a more parsimonious (and mainstream) framework for interpreting these results.

To answer this question, we first directly examined the relationship of shame-proneness and guilt-proneness to attributional style as measured by the Attributional Style Questionnaire in two studies of undergraduates (Tangney, Wagner, & Gramzow, 1992). The results across studies clearly indicated that shame-proneness is at least moderately linked to a depressogenic attributional style. Proneness to shame (and the unique variance in shame) was positively correlated with the tendency to make internal, stable, and global attributions for negative events, and negatively correlated with internal, stable, and (to a lesser extent) global attributions for positive events. The attributional style correlates of guilt-proneness were less consistent and did not reflect the expected pattern of results—that is, correlations with internal but unstable and specific attributions for negative events.

In both studies, shame-proneness was related to a depressogenic attributional style. Does a consideration of self-conscious affective style contribute to our understanding of depression, above and beyond that accounted for by attributional style? To answer this question, we conducted hierarchical regression analyses predicting BDI and SCL-90 depression scores from attributional style and affective style variables. In doing so, we forced in attributional style dimensions first, to provide the most conservative test of the incremental utility of proneness to shame. Results indicated that attributional style accounted for a significant portion of the variance in depression (7–14%, depending on the study and the measure used).

Shame-proneness and guilt-proneness were forced into the regression equations after attributional style variables. In each case, shame added important new information, accounting for an *additional* 8–15% of the variance in depression scores! These findings clearly indicate that the link between shame and depression is not solely due to attributional style. In fact, by including the affective component of shame (e.g., once attributional factors were controlled for) the proportion of variance predicted in depression was essentially doubled. Notably, guilt was largely irrelevant to depression.

IS THERE MALADAPTIVE GUILT?

In this chapter, we have described several lines of theory and a good deal of research suggesting that "pure" guilt, uncomplicated by shame, does not lead to psychological symptoms. In fact, such shame-free guilt appears to be quite adaptive, especially in regard to interpersonal issues. What, then, is the pathological guilt described by so many psychologists and psychotherapists? We agree that, in some significant instances, guilt can take a turn for the worse. The clinical literature frequently refers to a maladaptive guilt, characterized by chronic self-blame and obsessive rumination over an objectionable behavior.

We believe that guilt is most likely to be maladaptive when it becomes fused with shame. And it is the *shame* component that creates the problem. Imagine a guilt experience that begins with the thought, "Oh, look at what a horrible thing I have done," but which is then magnified and generalized to the self, "and aren't I a horrible person." Here there's a sequence from tension and remorse over a specific behavior to much more global self-directed feelings of contempt and disgust. In our view, it is the shame component of this sequence, not the guilt component, that poses a tortuous dilemma. Often, an objectionable behavior can be altered, the negative effects can be repaired, or at least one can offer a heartfelt apology. Even in cases where direct reparation or apology is not possible, one can resolve to do better in the future. For example, it may be impossible to directly apologize to a now-deceased parent, but one can consciously make an effort to be a more devoted family member with the living. In contrast, a self that is defective at its core is much more difficult to transform or amend. Attempts at reparation or atonement are apt to be seen as inadequate, as the self remains unworthy. Thus, shame—and, in turn, shame-fused guilt—offers little opportunity for redemption. In our view, it is guilt *with an overlay of shame* that is most likely to lead to the interminable rumination and self-castigation so often described in the clinical literature.

Our research results are quite consistent with this view. First, studies involving the SCAAI and TOSCA indicate considerable shared variance between shame and guilt; that is, it appears that many individuals are prone to experience both shame and guilt in response to negative events (see Chapter 3). Further, as shown in the tables in Appendix A (e.g., Tables A.2, A.3, and A.4), bivariate correlations involving guilt (i.e., correlations including that variance shared with shame) look somewhat similar to those involving shame. But when shame is factored out from guilt (e.g., when considering the guilt residuals), we see a very different pattern of results emerging. Proneness to shame-free guilt appears to be the more adaptive affective style across many different aspects of psychological functioning.

The notion of shame-fused guilt makes good theoretical sense. It matches our own clinical observations, and it is consistent with our empirical results. But still there's the possibility that some truly behavior-focused guilt reactions become problematic—lingering through our day-to-day existence, robbing us of our peace—*maybe* without that nefarious element of shame.

To find out more about maladaptive guilt, we recently turned to experts on the streets—or college students, in any event—and asked them about good guilt, bad guilt, and the difference between the two. Specifically, we asked 71 college students to think of one occasion when the feeling of guilt was on balance largely *negative*, when "you felt bad and couldn't shake the feeling, and not much good came of it." Students were also asked to think of one occasion when the feeling of guilt was on balance largely *positive*, when "you felt bad, but were about to work through the feeling and come to some reasonable resolution." Finally, we asked respondents to compare the two experiences and try to articulate what the critical difference between the two was.

The first notable finding is that students had *no difficulty* recalling positive guilt experiences. Of the 71 students, only 4 said they couldn't think of a positive one. In other words, the notion of an adaptive guilt experience was not in any way foreign to these students. They understood immediately what we were talking about. Note that these were not middle-aged respondents with extensive wisdom, life experience, and opportunities for reflection. These were largely 18-year-old college freshmen. Yet they already knew, from firsthand experience, that guilt can serve adaptive functions.

But they also knew about negative guilt experiences. Only two had trouble with that—another significant observation.

What were the critical differences between these "good" versus "bad" guilt experiences? In their summary statements, our students listed all sorts of idiosyncratic differences between the two events. But, as we read the descriptions of the events, the overwhelming single factor distinguishing between positive and negative guilt events had to do with making some positive change—either making reparation in some way or resolving to make changes for the future. These positive changes and intentions seemed to allow people to work through the feeling—to feel guilt, and then to put it to rest. And it was an absence of positive change that seemed to set the stage for the gnawing, repetitive guilt that just won't go away.

The difference was *striking*. Of the 65 pairs of narratives, 33 highlighted this difference between "good" and "bad" guilt experiences. One student wrote that, in the positive experience, "I felt good when it was resolved"; and, in the negative experience, "I never shook that feeling of guilt by resolving the situation." Another student wrote, "In the situation where my sister got in trouble, I was unwilling to set the record straight. With my friend, I was able to discuss the problem and come to a resolution."

In trying to identify factors that foster maladaptive guilt experiences, we may want to consider *mutability* of the situation: How readily are people able to repair or undo the harm that was caused? Some events may have particularly immutable and serious consequences (e.g., death of a neglected grandmother or killing a child through careless driving). These may pose real problems for the person because repair and resolution may be blocked.

But here we should emphasize that there are at least two major paths to resolution and redemption: one concerns reparation of the *consequences* of the focal past event; the other focuses on amending the *causes* of potential future events (see Arora, 1998). In their stories of resolved guilt events, students referred about equally to repair of consequences of past events and to changes to causes of potential future events. In fact, if anything, they referred more often to causes of future events. So, although it may not be possible to undo the consequences of a past event, an alternative route to salvation may lie in the future. People can try to right wrongs by turning over a new leaf so that a similar problem won't happen again. For example, one student felt guilty when he started dating the girl his best friend liked. One positive outcome of his feeling of guilt was that he "realized he should think about all the possible consequences before rushing into something." Another student was caught very drunk by her mother and her best friend's mother. As a result, she went to Alcoholics Anonymous (AA) and an alcohol abuse class to get help.

When are problematic unresolved guilt experiences likely to arise? One can imagine that both situational and personal factors come into play. As we noted, situations vary in how mutable the consequences are. Situations vary, too, in how well they lend themselves to future change. (For example, how likely is it that this sort of event will come up again? How mutable are the causes?) No doubt, there are also individual differences that render some people prone to maladaptive experiences of guilt. People with rigid, inflexible notions of what constitutes adequate "atonement" may be particularly vulnerable to ruminative, unproductive guilt reactions. For example, people who believe in "an eye for an eye" are apt to become stuck because they can't think of alternative ways of apologizing and undoing. Similarly, some individuals may have a limited ability to envision future-oriented solutions—ways of turning over a new leaf and righting the wrong so that a similar situation won't happen again. Others may be more creative in identifying ways of repairing or changing, thus navigating more favorable outcomes.

Finally, an important factor that may contribute to ruminative guilt experiences has to do with "misplaced" responsibility. People at times may have a tendency to take on "misplaced" responsibility, to feel personally responsible for events beyond their control. This intriguing idea, highlighted by Zahn-Waxler and Robinson (1995) and Ferguson et al. (1999; Ferguson & Eyre, 2001), fits well with the notion of mutability of the event. To the extent that one is, in fact, not responsible for some bad outcome, it may be especially difficult to repair damage (that you didn't do) or to make constructive changes for the future (since it wasn't your fault anyway).

DOES SHAME SERVE ANY ADAPTIVE FUNCTION?

A related issue concerns the potential positive functions of shame. Throughout this book we emphasize the dark side of shame, underscoring its negative consequences for psychological adjustment and for interpersonal behavior. An obvious question, then, is "Why do we have the capacity to experience this emotion anyway?" What adaptive purpose might it serve?

Several decades ago, Tomkins (1963) suggested that shame serves an adaptive function by regulating experiences of excessive interest and excitement (see also Nathanson, 1987a, 1987c; Schore, 1991). According to this view, at very early stages of development some mechanism is needed to dampen interest and excitement in the context of social interactions (especially vis-à-vis the mother). Feelings of shame arise when a child's bid for attention is rebuffed or when a significant social exchange is interrupted (e.g., when a mother is distracted). Thus, feelings of shame are thought to help the very young child disengage when it is appropriate to do so.

More prevalent is the widely held assumption that because shame is such a painful emotion, feelings of shame help people avoid wrongdoing (Barrett, 1995; Ferguson & Stegge, 1995; Zahn-Waxler & Robinson, 1995), decreasing the likelihood of transgression and impropriety. As discussed in the next chapter, there is surprisingly little evidence for this inhibitory function of shame. Moral behaviors of all sorts have been associated with the tendency to experience guilt *but not shame.*

It is possible that there are some circumstances in which more global, self-focused feelings of shame may be useful. No doubt, there *are* instances when individuals are faced with fundamental shortcomings of the self (moral or otherwise) that would best be corrected. The acute pain of shame may in some cases motivate productive soul-searching and revisions to one's priorities and values. The challenge is to engage in such introspection and self-repair without becoming sidetracked by defensive reactions (e.g., denial, externalization, and anger) so often experienced in conjunction with shame. Such a positive function of shame might ensue from private, self-generated experiences of shame as opposed to public, other-generated shame episodes. Perhaps non-shame-prone, high-ego-strength individuals with a solid sense of self may occasionally use shame constructively in the privacy of their own thoughts. But, for most people, the debilitating, ego-threatening nature of shame makes this impossible.

To our way of thinking, the relevant question may not be "What adaptive purpose might shame serve now?" but rather "What purpose might it have served at earlier stages of evolution?" We view shame as a primitive emotion that likely served a more adaptive function in the distant past, among ancestors whose cognitive processes were less sophisticated in the context of a much simpler human society. This is consistent with the sociobiological approach taken by Gilbert (1997), Fessler (1999), and others. Fessler, for example, describes a primitive form of shame—*protoshame*—as an early mechanism for communicating submission, thus affirming relative rank in the dominance hierarchy of early humans. Similarly, and reminiscent of Leary's (1989; Leary, Landel, & Patton, 1996) analysis of the appeasement functions of blushing and embarrassment (see also Keltner, 1995), Gilbert (1997) has discussed the appeasement functions of shame and humiliation displays, noting continuities across human and nonhuman primates. This perspective emphasizes the role of shame and embarrassment as a means of communicating one's acknowledgment of wrongdoing, thus diffusing anger and aggression. In a related fashion, the motivation to withdraw—so often a component of the shame experience—may be a useful response, interrupting potentially threatening social interactions until the shamed individual has a chance to regroup.

Humankind, however, has evolved not only in terms of physical characteristics but also in terms of emotional and cognitive complexity. With increasingly complex perspective-taking and attributional abilities, modern humans have the capacity to distinguish between self and behavior, to take another person's perspective, and to empathize with others' distress. Whereas early moral goals centered on reducing potentially lethal aggression, clarifying social rank, and enhancing conformity to social norms, modern morality centers on the ability to acknowledge one's wrongdoing, accept responsibility, and take reparative action. In this sense, guilt may be the moral emotion of the new millennium.

SUMMARY AND CONCLUSIONS

In this chapter, we focused on the implications of shame and guilt for people's psychological well-being. We reviewed a variety of theories regarding the role of shame and guilt in psychopathology and then examined the scientific research on this issue. Taken together, the literature strongly suggests that shame is the more problematic emotion, linked to a range of psychological symptoms. In contrast, "pure" guilt, uncomplicated by shame, does not lead to psychological symptoms and can, in fact, be quite adaptive. We closed with a discussion of how and when guilt might become "maladaptive." As researchers in the field move away from a black-or-white conceptualization of guilt (Bybee & Tangney, 1996), the next challenge is to clarify for whom and under what conditions guilt serves adaptive as opposed to maladaptive functions. Here, no doubt, both situational factors and individual differences come into play. In all likelihood, this will be a hot area of inquiry in the coming decade.

NOTES

1. Freud developed his theory of superego development with boys in mind. But he then encountered a few problems vis-à-vis the other 50% of the population. Little girls don't have penises, and so the threat of castration is a bit moot. Recognizing this dilemma, Freud (1924/1961c, 1925/1961b) engaged in some largely post hoc tinkering with his original theory to accommodate this fundamental anatomical difference. The result was a rather unparsimonious version of female moral development. But, rather than acknowledging that there was a weakness in the theory (in fairness, Freud recognized some difficulties in this area), Freud concluded that there was a weakness in the feminine superego. Freud (1925/1961b) surmised that because girls' fear of castration is not nearly as profound as that of boys, the subsequent defensive identification with the threatening paternal authority figure is neither as profound nor as complete in the case of females. Hence, the feminine superego is less solidly forged. Freud wrote, "I cannot evade the notion (though I hesitate to give it expression) that for women the level of what is ethically normal is different from what it is in men. Their superego is never so inexorable, so impersonal, so independent of its emotional origins as we require it to be in men" (Freud, 1925/1961b, p. 257). As it turns out, this is one portion of Freudian theory that has been soundly refuted by empirical research (for a review, see Tangney, 1994).
2. Actually, the parallels between feelings of guilt and behavioral self-blame are not as strong as they might at first appear. In the literature on moral emotions, feelings of guilt are typically experienced in response to bona fide failures or transgressions—events for which the individual is at least in part responsible. In contrast, in the behavioral self-blame literature, the focus is on reactions to traumatic events—events that typically involve little actual responsibility on the part of the "victim." In fact, the whole point of Janoff-Bulman's (1979) hypothesis regarding the adaptive effects of behavioral self-blame is that traumatic events pose a serious challenge to people's "assumptive world" (views of the world as a just place, where bad things don't happen to good people). The presumed advantage of behavioral self-blame is that it provides victims with a sense of control and a restored faith in a "just world."
3. One question that arises when we are interpreting null results involving part correlational analyses is whether there remains in the residual variable any meaningful variance beyond measurement error; that is, whether in partialing out the variance shared with shame, we have effectively partialed out all of guilt's reliable and valid variance. Results involving measures of other constructs, however, indicate that this is not the case. In previous studies employing the SCAAI and/or the TOSCA, guilt residuals (the unique variance in guilt) have shown consistent positive correlations with interpersonal empathy and a range of con-

structive responses to anger (see Chapters 5 and 6), and consistent negative correlations with externalization of blame, resentment toward others, and a hostile/ aggressive sense of humor (Gessner & Tangney, 1990; Tangney, 1990; Tangney, Wagner, Fletcher, & Gramzow, 1992; see also Chapter 6). Thus, the negligible correlations between indices of psychopathology and guilt residuals are not simply due to a restriction of valid variance in the guilt residual.

Chapter 8

THE BOTTOM LINE

Moral Emotions and Moral Behavior

In the domain of morality, the ultimate question comes down to people's behavior: bottom line, do moral emotions actually promote moral behavior and inhibit transgression? In the preceding chapters, we have examined the implications of shame and guilt for people's emotional and social well-being—empathy, anger, psychological symptoms, and self-regard. We have argued that guilt is, on balance, the more adaptive, "moral" emotion. We have described a number of ways in which shame can lead us in unhealthy or destructive directions. But when it comes down to *actions* generally considered as moral (helping, sacrificing, telling difficult truths) or immoral (lying, cheating, stealing), how useful are shame and guilt? Do shame and guilt both help people avoid "doing wrong"?

A not uncommon assumption is that because these are painful emotions, feelings of shame and guilt keep people "on the straight and narrow," decreasing the likelihood of transgression and impropriety. Here, we are on shakier ground because until recently little research has directly addressed the implications of moral emotions for moral behavior. We have a lot of data showing that shame-prone people are less empathic, more angry, and more distressed than their less shame-prone peers. But are they less likely to steal from their neighbor? Are they more likely to cheat on their spouse?

MORAL EMOTIONS, MORAL REASONING, AND MORAL BEHAVIOR

Even in the vast literature on moral reasoning, surprisingly few studies have actually examined people's *behavior.* Researchers interested in moral reasoning focus on how people *think* rather than how they *feel* in the face of moral dilemmas. Most notable is Kohlberg's (1969) cognitive-developmental theory of moral reasoning. Kohlberg proposed that people's thinking about moral issues progresses in stages, paralleling Piaget's (1952) more general theory of cognitive development. At the lowest levels of moral reasoning, people focus on concrete ideas of right and wrong (e.g., "That's the rule") and consequences for the self (e.g., "getting in trouble"). At successively higher levels of moral reasoning, the arguments become more complex and less egocentric, incorporating notions of community, justice, and reciprocity (e.g., "fairness for the common good"). Kohlberg (1969) uses a series of moral "dilemmas" to assess people's level of moral reasoning. For example, there's the classic dilemma faced by "Heinz," who must decide whether or not to steal a prohibitively expensive drug to save his dying wife. The issue isn't *what* people decide (steal vs. not steal), but *how* they decide. At lower levels of moral reasoning, a person might emphasize that stealing is against the rules or that Heinz might get caught and go to jail. At higher levels of moral reasoning, a person might also argue against stealing but draw on notions of fairness (someone else equally deserving would be deprived of the drug) or the need for order and justice in society.

How does level of moral reasoning relate to people's behavior? The very strong assumption among moral developmentalists is that people who reason at more sophisticated levels behave better, but the available evidence suggests only a modest link between moral thinking and moral action (Arnold, 1989; Blasi, 1980). Upon closer consideration, however, this modest relationship isn't all that surprising. As Blasi pointed out, in many instances there is no obvious correspondence between a given mode of moral reasoning and a particular behavioral choice. For example, altruistic behavior may result from reasoning at any level. A person might choose to help because "it's the rule" or out of appreciation for the needs of human society. By the same token, two individuals operating from the same moral cognitive level may behave in radically different ways, depending on the manner in which a situation in construed. It is possible to reason in a simple concrete fashion both that Heinz should steal and that he should not.

One criticism of Kohlberg's (1969) conceptualization and assessment of moral reasoning is its presumed bias against females. For many years, psychologists voiced concern that men reason at a higher moral developmental level than women on Kohlberg's Moral Judgment Interview. But Walker's (1984) comprehensive review of the empirical research on gender differences in moral reasoning concludes that there is actually little evidence for such gender differences in *level* of moral reasoning (see also Baumrind, 1986, and Walker, 1986). Rather, psychologists have increasingly focused on gender differences in the *nature* or substantive content of moral reasoning.

Along these lines, Gilligan (1982) convincingly argued that there are two different but equally legitimate bases for evaluating moral issues. Kohlberg (1969) emphasized an "ethic of justice" that focuses on rights and rules, and that emphasizes fairness, equality, and reciprocity. In contrast, Gilligan introduced the notion of an "ethic of care" that accentuates selflessness, interdependence, and responsibility in the context of relationships. She suggested that women are more inclined to reason about moral issues from this "ethic of care" perspective, whereas men are inclined to reason from a "justice" perspective. As stated by Tavris (1992), "Women feel the 'moral imperative' to care for others; men, to protect the rights of others" (p. 80). Considerable empirical evidence now supports Gilligan's assertion that women are inclined to rely more heavily than men on an ethic of care in their reasoning about moral dilemmas (Eisenberg, Fabes, & Shea, 1989; Gilligan & Attanucci, 1988; Skoe, Pratt, Matthews, & Curror, 1996; Skoe & Gooden, 1993; Soechting, Skoe, & Marcia, 1994; Stiller & Forrest, 1990; Wark & Krebs, 1996; White, 1994; White & Manolis, 1997).

A final drawback of the cognitive theories of moral development is that they lack any systematic consideration of moral emotion. Although Gilligan's description of the ethic of care implies some consideration of feelings of sympathy and concern, like Kohlberg's, hers is a theory of moral *reasoning*. The failure to consider moral emotion as an integral part of moral decision making and behavior is a major omission in our view for two reasons. First, issues of motivation, in general, are ignored. Second, there is a critical loss of information about potentially *compet-*

ing motives operative in a given situation (e.g., the other-oriented concern associated with empathy vs. self-related defensive processes associated with shame).

The research on moral reasoning and moral emotion has largely proceeded along independent lines. One notable exception is Eisenberg's (1986) work which presents a detailed analysis of the role of empathy in one important subset of moral thinking—prosocial reasoning. From Eisenberg's perspective, other-oriented empathy (or sympathy) is, by definition, a component of higher levels of prosocial reasoning. Empathically based prosocial reasoning has been associated with higher levels of altruistic helping behavior among both children and adults. However, virtually nothing is known about the link between more general aspects of (Kohlbergian) moral reasoning and moral emotional style (e.g., do empathic or guilt-prone individuals tend to reason at higher levels of moral thought?), and no research has sought to systematically integrate a range of moral cognitive and moral emotional factors in the study of moral behavior.

Moral decisions and moral behavior are presumably guided by three broad classes of factors: *moral standards*, *moral reasoning*, and *moral emotion*. Moral standards represent the individual's knowledge of culturally defined moral norms and conventions. As Blasi (1980) pointed out, there are very small individual differences in knowledge of accepted rules and norms beyond the early age of 7 or 8. For example, most people know that, barring extenuating circumstances, it is wrong to lie, cheat, or steal.

Naturally, people do on occasion lie, cheat, and steal, even though they know such behavior is wrong according to societal norms. Individual differences in both moral reasoning and moral emotion likely play a key role in determining people's actual moral choices and behavior in real life contexts. Moral reasoning involves thinking through the implications of alternative behaviors in terms of moral principles. Not infrequently, people are faced with competing moral considerations (as in Kohlberg's "Heinz" dilemma), and it is here that individual differences in moral developmental level presumably come into play. But perhaps more important is people's capacity for moral emotions. Moral emotions provide immediate punishment (or reinforcement) of behavior. Moreover, people can *anticipate* their likely emotional reactions (e.g., guilt) as they consider behavioral alternatives. It is our guess that individual differences in the capacity to experience these emotions—guilt, shame, and empathy—should be more directly tied to behavior than individual differences in the level of reasoning.

MORAL EMOTION AND MORAL BEHAVIOR: IS THERE EVIDENCE FOR A LINK?

Scientists have yet to examine the relative importance of moral reasoning and moral emotion in shaping people's moral behavior. Indeed, moral reasoning aside, only a few studies have even examined the relationship between moral emotions and moral behavior.

In one study (Tangney, 1994), we examined the relationship of individual differences in proneness to shame and guilt to self-reported moral behavior (assessed by the Conventional Morality Scale; Tooke & Ickes, 1988). We found that self-reported moral behaviors were substantially positively correlated with proneness to guilt but unrelated to proneness to shame. For example, compared to their less-guilt-prone peers, guilt-prone individuals were more likely to endorse such items as "I would not steal something I needed, even if I were sure I could get away with it," "I will not take advantage of other people, even when it's clear that they are trying to take advantage of me," and "Morality and ethics don't really concern me" (reversed). In other words, results from this study suggest that guilt *but not shame* helps people choose the "moral paths" in life.

The most direct evidence linking moral emotions with moral behavior comes from our ongoing Longitudinal Family Study of moral emotions. In this study, 380 index children, their parents, and their grandparents were initially studied when index children were in the fifth grade. Children were recruited from public schools in an ethnically and socioeconomically diverse suburb of Washington, DC (60% of the sample is white, 31% black, and 9% other). Most children generally came from low- to moderate-income families. The typical parents had attained a high school education. Eight years later, we gathered a third panel of data that included an in-depth social and clinical history interview of index children at ages 18–19. Preliminary analyses show that moral emotional style in the fifth grade predicts critical "bottom line" behaviors in young adulthood (ages 18–19), including the following:

- Drug and alcohol use
- Risky sexual behavior

- Involvement with the criminal justice system (arrests, convictions, incarceration)
- Suicide attempts
- High school suspension
- Community service involvement

More specifically, shame-proneness assessed in the fifth grade predicted later high school suspension, drug use of various kinds (amphetamines, depressants, hallucinogens, heroin), and suicide attempts. Relative to their less shame-prone peers, shame-prone children were less likely to apply to college or engage in community service.

In contrast, relative to less guilt-prone children, guilt-prone fifth graders were more likely to later apply to college and do community service. They were less likely to make suicide attempts, to use heroin, and to drive under the influence of alcohol or drugs, and they began drinking at a later age. Guilt-prone fifth graders were less likely to be arrested, convicted, and incarcerated. In adolescence they had fewer sexual partners and were more likely to practice "safe sex" and use birth control.

These links between early moral emotional style and subsequent behavioral adjustment remained robust, even when we controlled for family income and mothers' education. Thus, this is not simply an effect of socioeconomic status. Moreover, these findings held even when controlling for children's anger at time 1 (fifth grade). The robustness with respect to time 1 anger is especially impressive, given that early indices of anger and aggression are some of the most important predictors of later criminal activity and other behavioral maladjustment (Huesmann, Eron, Lefkowitz, & Walder, 1984).

Paralleling these results from our longitudinal study of moral emotions, L. R. Huesmann (personal communication, February 2, 2001) has observed a differential relationship of children's shame and guilt with later behavioral adjustment. In his long-term longitudinal study of 335 children, Huesmann found that parents' reports of children's guilt at age 8 were a significant negative predictor of number of arrests and episodes of serious physical aggression 22 *years later*, when the children had reached age 30. In contrast, feelings of shame did not appear to serve as a deterrent for later aggression and criminal activity. Parents' reports of children's shame at age 8 showed positive, nonsignificant links to number of arrests and serious physical aggression at age 30.

GUILT, NOT SHAME, IS THE
MORAL EMOTION OF CHOICE

Our longitudinal study provides the first solid empirical findings linking shame and guilt to bottom line "moral" and "immoral" behaviors.
The pattern is pretty clear cut: guilt is good; shame is bad.

The link between hard drug use and the propensity for shame
about the self is consistent with the clinical literature on addictions
(Bradshaw, 1988; Fossum & Mason, 1986; Potter-Efron, 1989). Substance abuse experts have suggested that problematic alcohol and drug
use develop as a misguided, maladaptive style of coping with dysfunctional family environments. For example, in discussing the development of maladaptive coping styles (such as substance abuse), Linehan
(1993a, 1993b) has described an "invalidating" family environment in
which family members' emotional reactions are routinely ignored, dis-
counted, or belittled. Such an environment only serves to turn up the
emotional volume—particularly negative emotions such as anger,
shame, and loneliness. Some individuals respond by using alcohol and/
or drugs to dampen their distressing emotions. Unfortunately, it's a
quick but fleeting "fix." Although drugs or alcohol can numb the pain
in the short run, what often ensues is a destructive cycle of addiction
and shame. As Potter-Efron (1989) observed, "Individuals who get
caught in this pattern often drink in order to escape their shame, only to
find that eventually they feel even more shame because they have been
drinking out of control" (p. 128). Indeed, in addition to our results
from the Longitudinal Family Study, described earlier, empirical studies
support the link between shame and substance abuse (O'Connor, Berry,
Inaba, & Weiss, 1994), dysfunctional family environments (Pulakos,
1996), and codependent characteristics (Wells, Glickauf-Hughes, &
Jones, 1999, but see Jones & Zelewski, 1994).

It's easy to imagine how this cycle of shame can lead to a profound
sense of hopelessness and despair. And, in fact, our finding of a link between shame and suicide is consistent with results from studies of college students (Hastings, Northman, & Tangney, 2000; Lester, 1998) and
with the theories and observations of leading experts in the field of suicide (Durkheim, 1966; Hassan, 1995; Scheff, 1997; Schneidman, 1968),
who have long noted the significance of shame in the dynamics of
suicidality. For example, in two independent studies of 254 and 230 undergraduates, Hastings et al. (2000) found that a dispositional tendency
to experience shame across a range of situations was reliably linked to
suicidal ideation as well as to overall depression scores, as measured by

the BDI and SCL-90. The findings regarding guilt were markedly different. People who were prone to "shame-free" guilt showed no vulnerability to depression and, if anything, were less inclined toward suicidal thoughts and behaviors than their peers.

In addition, studies investigating precipitants or causes of suicide have identified feelings of shame as triggers of suicide. Using data from coroners' case files, Hassan (1995) found that the most common cause of suicide was "a sense of failure in life." Hassan defined this category as a history of many things "going wrong" that were associated with a sense of failure and giving up on life. Many of the examples given (i.e., a combination of factors such as loss of employment, loss of face, failure to meet family obligations, and failure in a business or profession) are commonly associated with significant feelings of shame or guilt. Similar results were observed in an earlier study of 400 completed suicides in Singapore (Hassan, 1980). Thus, feelings of shame may be of central importance in understanding suicidal behavior.

We should emphasize that in our Longitudinal Family Study, no apparent benefit was derived from the pain of shame. There was no evidence that shame inhibits problematic behaviors. The propensity for shame does not deter young people from engaging in criminal activities; it does not deter them from unsafe sex practices; it does not foster responsible driving habits; and in fact it seems to *inhibit* constructive involvement in community service.

Guilt, on the other hand, seems to be a powerful moral emotional factor. People who have the capacity to feel guilt about specific behaviors are *less* likely than their non-guilt-prone peers to engage in destructive, impulsive, and/or criminal activities. They have sex with fewer partners and are more likely to use protection. They are more likely to drive responsibly, to apply to college, and to actively contribute to the community.

In short, given a choice, most parents would prefer to raise a guilt-prone child. The next chapter examines how these moral emotional styles develop. What factors help shape children's development of a healthy, constructive capacity for guilt as opposed to a propensity for shame about the self?

SUMMARY AND CONCLUSIONS

Do moral emotions guide moral behavior? The answer from two studies is "Yes," but it is not simply a case of "more is better." Guilt about specific behaviors appears to steer people in a moral direction—fostering constructive, responsible behavior in many critical domains. Shame, in contrast, does little to inhibit immoral action. Instead, painful feelings of shame seem to promote self-destructive behaviors (hard drug use, suicide) that can be viewed as misguided attempts to dampen or escape this most punitive moral emotion.

Chapter 9

SHAME AND GUILT
ACROSS THE LIFESPAN

The Development of Moral Emotions

This chapter addresses two broad questions related to the development of moral emotions. The first question focuses on normative developmental changes in how people experience shame and guilt. Is a 6-year-old's shame experience the same as that of a 60-year-old? Does the nature, meaning, and function of moral emotions change across the lifespan? The second question focuses on individual differences in shame-proneness and guilt-proneness. Adolescents may be more or less shame-prone than middle-aged adults, but *within* a given age group there are substantial individual differences in the proneness to moral emotions. Where do these differences come from? What biological and environmental factors shape a child's emerging moral emotional style?

For many readers, the question about individual differences is of greatest interest. A fundamental issue facing parents, teachers, and psychologists alike is how to help children develop an internalized core sense of morality—an enduring motivation to "do the right thing." But before examining individual differences, it's useful to have an understanding of when the capacity to experience various moral emotions emerges and how normative experiences of shame, guilt, and empathy change with age.

THE EXPERIENCE OF MORAL EMOTIONS ACROSS
THE LIFESPAN: NORMATIVE DEVELOPMENTAL CHANGES

Most of the studies we have discussed in this book were conducted on samples of college students and adults. In fact, much of what we know about these "moral" emotions is from an adult perspective. How far can these results be generalized to younger individuals? Do children and adolescents experience shame and guilt in much the same way as their parents and grandparents do? Do these emotions play the same role in regulating children's behavior in interpersonal settings, shaping them into "moral" children, and later in the same way into "moral" adults?

Most developmental psychologists would agree: it is extremely unlikely that the nature and functions of "self-conscious" emotions, such as shame and guilt, remain the same across the lifespan. In contrast to the "basic" emotions (e.g., anger, fear, joy), which emerge very early in life, shame and guilt are considered more developmentally advanced. These "secondary" or "derived" emotions emerge later and hinge on two cognitive milestones: (1) a clear recognition of the self as separate from others, and (2) the development of standards against which the self and/or one's behavior is evaluated (M. Lewis, Sullivan, Stanger, & Weiss, 1989; Fischer & Tangney, 1995). When bad things happen, many different types of negative emotions are possible—for example, sadness, disappointment, frustration, or anger. But feelings of shame and guilt typically arise from a recognition of one's *own* negative attributes or negative behaviors, attributes and behaviors that fail to match up to some internally or externally imposed standard. Even when we feel shame due to another person's behavior, that person is almost invariably someone with whom we are closely affiliated or identified (e.g., a family member, friend, or colleague closely associated with the self). We experience shame because that person is part of our self-definition.

In short, self-conscious emotions are about the self; they require a concept of self and a set of standards as a point of comparison. In addition, in the special case of guilt, a third ability is required. It is necessary to make a clear distinction between self and behavior in order to experience guilt about specific behaviors, separate from shame about the self.

Children aren't born with the ability to experience shame and guilt. None of these cognitive abilities (recognition of the self, standards, distinction between self and behavior) is present at birth. These cognitive milestones emerge in childhood, first as a glimmer of an ability, and later in development as increasingly complex and elaborated capacities.

Changes in Conceptions of the Self

A person's conception of self—of who he or she is—shifts dramatically from early childhood into adulthood (Damon & Hart, 1982). In turn, these changes undoubtedly shape and define the nature of "self-conscious" emotions (see Mascolo & Fischer, 1995). Developmental psychologists generally agree that children are not born with a sense of self. The notion of a "self" distinct from others appears to emerge in the second year of life. And it is at this point in the developmental process that signs of self-conscious emotions first appear. For example, in a series of studies, M. Lewis et al. (1989) demonstrated that very young children first show signs of embarrassment (smiling coupled with gaze aversion, touching the face, etc.) in embarrassing situations between 15 and 24 months. Not coincidentally, this is the same phase of development in which a rudimentary sense of self emerges. Researchers assess self-recognition by surreptitiously putting rouge on a child's nose and subsequently observing the child's behavior when faced with a mirror (Amsterdam, 1972; Bertenthal & Fischer, 1978). Prior to 15 months, children may look with interest at "the red nose in the mirror," but they don't seem to connect the image with themselves. Between 15 and 24 months, however, children begin to show signs of self-recognition—spontaneously touching or wiping *their* rouged nose. M. Lewis et al. (1989) not only demonstrated that embarrassment and self-recognition on the "rouge" task emerge within the same developmental phase. *Within* the 15- to 24-month span of development, children who show self-recognition (in the "rouge" test) are the very same children who display signs of embarrassment in an unrelated task. Kids who don't yet recognize the self, don't yet show embarrassment. M. Lewis and colleagues' (1989) results are consistent with the notion that a recognized self is a *prerequisite* for emotions such as embarrassment, shame, guilt, and pride.

Certainly, a person's conception of self continues to evolve considerably beyond age 15 months (Damon & Hart, 1982). Children move from a self defined by fairly concrete, often observable characteristics (e.g., "I am a girl"; "I am tall") to a self defined by current activities and involvements ("I am a swimmer"; "I am a hockey player"), and then to a self constructed by more enduring patterns of behavior ("I am nice to my friends"; "I do well at school"). Still later, such characteristics are organized and integrated into a coherent self-identity, forged of abstract, sophisticated personality traits ("I am a generous, creative, shy person"). Thus, there are dramatic changes in the "self" that one is conscious of, or that one evaluates, in shame or guilt experiences.

Changes in the Structure of Moral Standards and the Nature of Transgressions

There are substantial age-related shifts, too, in the structure of children's moral standards. A rudimentary sense of right and wrong can be seen in toddlers' social interactions with their mothers (Smetana, 1989), but across the preschool years the domain of moral judgments expands to include more events and take into account more facets of the events. By about age 4, children have distinct notions about transgressions' seriousness, punishability, and contingency on rules, and they can reliably distinguish between moral transgressions and violations of social convention (Smetana, Schlagman, & Adams, 1993).

In a study of children's and adults' descriptions of personal shame and guilt experiences (Tangney et al., 1994), we examined age differences in the content, structure, and interpersonal focus of emotion-eliciting events. The most obvious age differences were in the specific content of the emotion-eliciting situations. This undoubtedly reflects the differential everyday experiences encountered by children and adults. For example, sex, infidelity, and the breakup of a romance were cited exclusively by adults; children were much more likely to mention disobeying parents, damaging objects, and accomplishments at a hobby or sport. In addition, however, there were developmental differences in the number of concrete versus abstract themes mentioned by respondents, consistent with Williams and Bybee's (1994) developmental analysis of guilt events. Williams and Bybee found that adolescents were more likely than children to mention guilt over inaction, neglect of responsibilities, and failure to attain ideals. Children are more inclined to focus on concrete, observable acts, such as hitting a sibling or breaking a toy, as opposed to adolescents who are able to recognize less visible failures and transgressions that may transcend time and place.

There are also important developmental changes in the internalization of rules and standards. That is, the events that elicit shame and guilt among children become increasingly internalized and self-relevant with age. Harris (1989) observed that, between the ages of 5 and 8, children progress from a narrow focus on the *outcome* of an action (e.g., do they view the outcome as good or bad, regardless of any personal responsibility on the part of the child?), to a consideration of *others' reac-*

tions to a behavior (e.g., parental approval or disapproval). Still later, children's reactions become even more sophisticated, including a consideration of their *own reaction* (approval or disapproval) to their behavior (see also Harter & Whitesell, 1989). Children's norms and standards continue to become more internalized in later childhood and adolescence. For example, in characterizing shame and guilt experiences, younger children (about age 8) are more likely to focus on *other* people's evaluations and reactions, compared to older children (about age 11). Older children seem to rely more on their *own* standards in evaluating their behavior (Ferguson et al., 1991).

In contrast, Tangney et al. (1994) found no evidence for a main effect of age on internalization. In this study, we conceptualized "internalization" as the degree to which feelings of shame and guilt were contingent on other people's involvement in shame- and guilt-eliciting events. Surprisingly, the emotion experiences of adult respondents were no more internalized or "autonomous" than those of children (ages 8–12). In their descriptions of shame, guilt, and pride, adults were just as likely as children to refer to an audience in their account of the events. Similarly, there were no overall age differences in the number of people present, in the degree to which others were *aware* of the respondent's behavior, or in the extent to which respondents were concerned with others' evaluation of the self.

There was, however, an intriguing *interaction* between age and emotion in predicting audience concerns. In general, these audience dimensions varied little across the three emotions for children. But among adults a much more differentiated picture emerged, especially when we considered the nature of respondents' interpersonal concerns. Adults were more concerned with others' evaluation in shame and pride situations, and differentially more concerned with their effect on others in guilt situations. Children's interpersonal focus was fairly uniform across the three emotions, suggesting significant developmental changes, beyond middle childhood, in the degree to which shame and guilt become distinct self-conscious emotions.

Changes in the Degree to Which Shame and Guilt Are Distinct Emotions

Developmental research suggests that the capacity to experience guilt and shame as distinct emotions develops gradually with age. Although Barrett et al. (1993) have shown that toddlers exhibit distinct *behavioral responses* to transgression (hiding vs. amending), these individual differences in behavior could be attributed to temperament, socialization, and a host of other factors. Given an 18-month-old's rudimentary sense of self, it seems unlikely that he or she could experience a well-articulated feeling of guilt (about a specific behavior), distinct from shame (about the self). Shame and guilt are "attribution-dependent emotions" (Ferguson & Rule, 1983; Ferguson & Stegge, 1995) that hinge not only on evaluations of the *valence* of the event but also on fairly complex evaluations of the *causes* of that event. For example, feelings of shame are most likely to arise from internal, stable, and global attributions for negative events (i.e., a bad self). Feelings of guilt are most likely to arise from internal but fairly unstable and specific attributions for negative events (i.e., a bad behavior).

Children are not very adept at making complex attributions until well into middle childhood. For example, before age 8, children largely focus on the valence of an event's outcome (was it good or bad?), not the cause of the event (was it my fault or someone else's?; P. L. Harris, 1989). Also at about age 8, children begin to distinguish between enduring characteristics of the self and more transient types of behaviors—for example, making a meaningful distinction between attributions to ability (enduring characteristics) and attributions to effort (more unstable, volitional factors; Nicholls, 1978).

Not surprisingly, research on children's understanding of shame and guilt has shown that children don't reliably distinguish between these two "attribution-dependent" emotions until middle childhood. At ages 5 to 6, children are unable to describe events that would elicit shame and guilt (P. L. Harris, Olthof, Terwogt, & Hardman, 1987). Similarly, Denham and Couchaud (1991) observed that very young children typically describe a vague sort of feeling "bad" in varying negative situations, including transgressions and failure, but are unable to articulate differentiated shame and guilt experiences. This is likely due to limited language ability as well as to children's relatively unsophisticated causal attributions.

By age 8, when children begin to distinguish between stable and unstable attributions (e.g., attributions to behavior vs. attributions to character), notable differences emerge in children's reports of shame and guilt experiences (Ferguson et al., 1990a, 1990b, 1991). The majority of children of this age, for example, understood the special connection between guilt and reparative behavior and the connection between shame and denial. In our own research, we found few reliable differences in 8- to 12-year-old children's phenomenological ratings of personal shame and guilt experiences, but a qualitative analysis of their narrative accounts revealed some important differences between descriptions of shame- and guilt-eliciting events (Tangney et al., 1994). Like adults, children conveyed more other-oriented empathy and perspective taking in their descriptions of guilt events, and there were some differences in the types of events cited in connection with emotions (although, as in previous studies [e.g., Tangney, 1992], there were clearly more similarities than differences in the types of events that give rise to feelings of shame and guilt). But adults' narrative accounts showed even more pronounced phenomenological differences between shame and guilt, indicating that, beyond childhood, shame and guilt continue to evolve as distinct affective experiences.

Changes in Propensity to Experience Shame and Guilt

Thus far, we have been considering developmental differences in the *nature* of the shame and guilt experience. When does the capacity to experience these moral emotions emerge? Are there differences, especially in the first 8–10 years of life, in what shame and guilt feel like?—in how children understand these emotions?

A second set of questions concern developmental differences in the *propensity* to experience shame and guilt. Once the capacity to experience these distinct moral emotions has developed (i.e., about ages 8–10), are there age-related changes in people's susceptibility to these emotions? Are 20-year-olds just as shame-prone as 60-year-olds? In several studies of college students and adults, we found a modest decline in proneness to shame from early to middle adulthood. More recent analyses of our intergenerational family study, however, indicate that, if anything, children's grandparents are more shame-prone than the children's parents.

INDIVIDUAL DIFFERENCES IN MORAL EMOTIONAL STYLE

So far, we have been discussing normative developmental differences in the experience of moral emotions across the lifespan: in general, how is the experience of a 60-year-old different from that of a 6-year-old? There are, however, individual differences in the degree to which people are *prone* to either shame or guilt, or both. Within a given age group, say, adolescents, some people are more prone to shame and some more prone to guilt. That is, in the face of similar failures and transgressions, some 16-year-olds feel guilt (about a specific behavior) whereas others feel shame (about the entire self).

Results from our ongoing longitudinal study indicate that these individual differences in proneness to shame and guilt are remarkably stable from middle childhood into early adulthood. (See Table A.5 in Appendix A for the stabilities of children's proneness to shame and guilt over an 8-year period.) Shame-proneness and guilt-proneness at age 10 (as assessed by the TOSCA-C) was quite predictive of shame-proneness and guilt-proneness at age 12 (as assessed by the TOSCA-A). In turn, shame-proneness and guilt-proneness at age 12 was quite predictive of shame-proneness and guilt-proneness at age 18 (again assessed with the TOSCA-A). Finally, shame- and guilt-proneness were remarkably stable across the 8-year period. These are quite stable affective dispositions, especially when we consider the length of time between assessments, the phase of development under consideration (there is a great deal going on during that transition through adolescence), and the fact that we used two different measures of shame- and guilt-proneness. Not surprisingly, stabilities were even higher among the children's parents and grandparents over the same period of time (see Table A.6 in Appendix A for more detail). A person's relative position among his or her peers remains fairly stable. That is, 10-year-olds who are more shame-prone than their classmates in fifth grade are still likely, 8 years later, to be more shame-prone than their high school peers.

As described in detail throughout this book, shame-proneness and guilt-proneness are individual differences that *matter.* For the child, these individual differences have far-reaching implications for life at home, in the classroom, and on the playground. In adolescence and adulthood, too, proneness to shame and guilt are linked to fundamental aspects of people's psychological and social well-being. We still must answer the $100,000 question: Where do these differences in moral emotional style come from? or How do these individual differences in proneness to shame and guilt develop?

HOW DO INDIVIDUAL DIFFERENCES IN MORAL EMOTIONAL STYLES DEVELOP?

The family is an obvious first place to look. Emphasizing the importance of the family, researchers have noted intergenerational continuities in attachment (Benoit & Parker, 1994), depression (Whitbeck et al.,

1992), aggression (Widom, 1987, 1989), and harsh parenting (Simons, Whitbeck, Conger, & Wu, 1991). Aggressive parents tend to have aggressive children. Securely attached parents tend to have securely attached children. Harsh parents raise children who become harsh parents. Both genetic and environmental (socialization) factors undoubtedly contribute to these intergenerational links.

Are there similar intergenerational continuities in moral emotional style as well? Do families—via genetics or socialization or both—play a key role in shaping children's propensity to experience moral emotions?

In terms of socialization, the family might be influential in at least three ways (see Figure 9.1): First, parents' affective styles may directly influence those of their children. In their day-to-day interactions, parents provide powerful models for their children simply by how they themselves react to negative events. For example, a child may repeatedly observe Mom reacting with shame when faced with negative interpersonal exchanges. The mother may display a shrinking posture and downcast eyes. She may verbalize shame-related self-statements (e.g., "God, I'm so stupid!") and attempt to escape from shame-inducing situations. In this way, over the course of repeated daily events, the child may learn that a particular pattern of emotional, cognitive, and behavioral responses is appropriate in certain kinds of situations. To the degree that such direct modeling occurs, one would expect a direct link between parents' affective styles and those of their children. Second, family members' affective styles may be shaped by more general aspects of the family environment. Current work on family systems and on

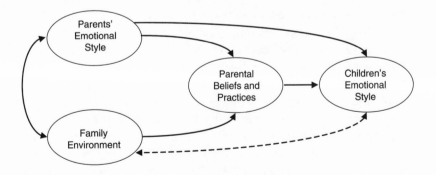

FIGURE 9.1. Socialization of shame and guilt.

codependence, for example (Bradshaw, 1988; Fossum & Mason, 1986), describes a *shame-based* family system—a system characterized by maladaptive patterns of communication and by the extremes of family conflict and/or enmeshment. From this perspective, intergenerational continuities would arise not simply from direct modeling but from more general interactions within the family system. And research confirms a relationship between shame and substance abuse (O'Connor et al., 1994), dysfunctional family environments (Pulakos, 1996), and codependent characteristics (Wells et al., 1999; but see Jones & Zelewski, 1994). Third, rather than (or in addition to) a direct link between parents' and children's emotional styles, certain parenting practices may play a crucial mediating role. Parental beliefs and practices may have the most direct impact on the development of children's emotional styles (see Figure 9.1). These parenting practices may be determined in part by aspects of the family environment and in part by affective characteristics of the parents. One would still expect intergenerational continuities in moral emotional style, but according to this view it is the parenting beliefs and practices that are most proximal to the development of children's shame and guilt.

EMPIRICAL RESEARCH ON THE DEVELOPMENT OF INDIVIDUAL DIFFERENCES IN MORAL EMOTIONAL STYLE: WHAT DOES THE EVIDENCE SHOW?

Intergenerational Continuities and Discontinuities in Proneness to Shame and Guilt

Do shame-prone parents have shame-prone children? To what degree is there a correspondence between the moral emotional styles of parents and children? To answer these questions, we have been conducting a longitudinal study of 380 index children, their parents, and their grandparents. This intergenerational sample was initially studied in 1990 (Panel 1), when the index children were in the fifth grade. Children were recruited from nine public elementary schools in an ethnically and socioeconomically diverse community in suburban Washington, DC.

Our initial analysis of the Panel 1 (fifth grade) data showed only modest evidence of direct transmission of shame and guilt across the generations (Tangney et al., 1991). These initial analyses, however, focused on birth fathers. Because our theoretical focus is on parental *socialization* of children's moral emotional styles, our focus should be on the "psychological" fathers. We subsequently reanalyzed the data using only "psychological" fathers.[1]

The focus on psychological fathers sharpened the results, consistently pointing to fathers as important in the development of an adaptive, guilt-prone style. Fathers' proneness to guilt was significantly related to sons' guilt, and there was a parallel relationship between fathers' and both paternal grandparents' guilt. There was also a link between mothers' and maternal grandfathers' guilt. But it is notable that most findings for females (in contrast to males) failed to replicate across the generations.

How might this link between the moral emotional styles of fathers and sons develop in the course of day-to-day family life? Developmental psychologists emphasize that much important "social learning" occurs in the family context. Sons observe as their fathers fail or transgress, experience guilt, and respond with focused reparative action. For example, imagine a situation in which Dad forgets his wedding anniversary, coming home clueless and empty handed. Mom reacts with obvious disappointment. Feeling guilty, Dad apologizes for his error, acknowledges his wife's disappointment, and makes plans for special night out later in the week. He then orders in dinner from his wife's favorite Chinese restaurant, joking with his son, "I hope you're learning from this— Remember those anniversaries! And when you don't, own up, give her a hug, and order out!"

In short, parents have the opportunity to exert a powerful influence on how their children feel and respond to the inevitable errors and transgressions of daily life. We hope to have much more to say about intergenerational patterns in moral emotional style from further follow-up and analysis of our ongoing intergenerational family study. But for now we can tentatively conclude that, in the area of moral emotional style, there is a special link between fathers and sons, especially when considering guilt. In contrast, there do not appear to be clear intergenerational continuities between mothers and daughters.

Effects of Parenting Style on Moral Emotional Development

In addition to direct modeling, children's moral affective styles may be shaped by certain parenting practices. Although several researchers have examined the link between parenting behavior and moral emotional development, there are some ambiguities in this literature because of inconsistencies in distinguishing between shame and guilt.

Some of the foremost research on the emotional development of young children focuses on guilt without considering shame as a distinct emotional experience. As a consequence, guilt is often operationalized in ways that incorporate both shame and guilt experiences. For example, in their study of guilt among children of depressed and nondepressed mothers, Zahn-Waxler et al. (1990) operationalized guilt by coding children's transgression stories for expressions of remorse, self-punishment, reparation, apology, and blameworthiness. Included were shame-like responses such as "She feels like a bad girl." A second measure of guilt, based on structured psychiatric interviews, was designed to assess "self-blame or self-attributions of responsibility for negative events" including evidence of "feeling ashamed." Similarly, in Kochanska's (1991, 1994) otherwise impressive work on the interaction between socialization and temperament in the development of conscience, no distinction is made between shame and guilt. Both shame and guilt are included under the rubric of conscience.

Throughout this book, we have presented evidence from diverse domains that shame and guilt are distinct emotions with very different implications for psychological adjustment and social behavior. Thus the types of parenting behaviors that differentially predict children's shame versus guilt are of special interest. Studies that combine shame- and guilt-related items into a single index of "conscience" or "guilt" are of limited use in this regard.

In recent years, several investigators have made an explicit distinction between shame and guilt. Results provide some initial support for the notion that parental beliefs and practices are an important component of the socialization of moral emotions. In a study of 39 children 5–12 years old, Ferguson and Stegge (1995) found that children's guilt was associated with parents' reports of induction (i.e., focusing the child's attention on the emotional reactions of others) and parental anger in negative situations, whereas children's shame was associated with parental hostility, little recognition of positive outcomes, and a lack of discipline. Similarly, in two independent studies drawing on observations of parental behavior, Alessandri and Lewis (1993, 1996) found that mothers' negative comments about the child's performance was correlated with children's shame reactions during laboratory tasks. In studies of adults' retrospective reports of their parents' behavior, shame-proneness in adulthood was associated with recalled parental putdowns and shaming (Gilbert, Allan, & Goss, 1996), recalled parental protectiveness and lack of parental care (Lutwak & Ferrari, 1997), harsh and inconsistent parenting (Chandler-Holtz, 1999), parentification (i.e., the child being placed in a parental role; Wells & Jones, 2000), and recalled emotional abusiveness (Hoglund & Nicholas, 1995). Guilt-proneness, in contrast, has been associated with recall of inductive parental strategies (Abell & Gecas, 1997).

In our initial analyses of the intergenerational family study, we found no consistent relationship between parents' reports of their parenting attitudes (Block Childrearing Practices Report) and children's moral emotional style. However, conventional parenting inventories have been criticized for assessing attitudes that are too broad to be meaningfully related to actual parental behaviors and for presenting items that are devoid of specific contexts (Holden & Edwards, 1989). In particular, existing parenting measures, like the Block, do not address specific and often subtle parental behaviors thought to be relevant to the socialization of shame, guilt, and empathy.

To fill this gap, K. L. Rosenberg, Tangney, Denham, Leonard, and Widmaier (1994a, 1994b) developed a new set of parenting measures that focus on much more specific types of disciplinary strategies than the global parenting styles typically assessed by available measures. The Socialization of Moral Affect Inventories (SOMAs) were developed to assess specifically parental behaviors that are theoretically relevant to the socialization of shame, guilt, and empathy. These dimensions include the following: Love Withdrawal; Power Assertion (including corporal punishment); Victim-Focused Induction (where the focus of the induction is on the feelings and consequences for the victim); Parent-Focused Induction (where the focus of the induction is on the feelings and consequences for the parent); Teaching Reparation; Behavior-Focused Responses, both positive and negative; Person-Focused Responses—positive or negative evaluations; Neglect/Ignoring; Public Humiliation; Conditional Approval; and Disgust/Teasing/Contempt.

A key goal of K. L. Rosenberg's (1998) study was to examine the relationship of children's shame-proneness and guilt-proneness to SOMA-assessed parental behaviors theorized to be influential in the development of these styles. For example, it was expected that parenting behaviors that focused on the child as a person, rather than on the child's behavior, would be associated with shame-proneness in children. It was also expected that parenting behaviors that focused on the child's specific behavior and ways to "fix" any damage or harm caused by this behavior would be associated with children's guilt-proneness.

Results were in the predicted directions, primarily when considering children's perceptions of parental behavior (SOMA-C). Guilt-prone children reported that their parents were more likely to use behavior-focused messages and induction when disciplining them. Parents of guilt-prone children were less likely to ignore, express disgust at, or tease their children, and such parents tend not to use person-focused disciplinary messages. Fathers' love withdrawal was also negatively correlated with children's guilt-proneness. Similar but weaker results emerged from parents' self-reports. Parental self-reports of power assertion, disgust, and teasing were inversely correlated with children's proneness to guilt.

In contrast, shame-prone children reported that their parents were more likely to use person-focused disciplinary messages, express disgust, tease, communicate conditional approval, and use love withdrawal techniques. In addition, shame-proneness was associated with fathers' power assertion and mothers' use of public humiliation.

Parents' self-reports of disciplinary behavior were largely unrelated to children's shame-proneness, although parents' reports of their behavior were correlated with *their* own tendencies to experience shame and guilt.

In short, while there is some evidence that parenting practices affect children's moral emotional style, in both concurrent and retrospective studies, perceptions of parents' behavior seem to be particularly important in the development of shame- and guilt-proneness in children.

How Is Religious Background Related to the Propensity to Experience Shame and Guilt?

"Were you raised Catholic?" This is one of the most common questions people ask when they find out that we study shame and guilt.[2] It is commonly assumed that some religions are more "guilt-inducing" than others. Our culture is rife with jokes about "Catholic guilt" and the classic "guilt-inducing Jewish mother." As it turns out, religion doesn't matter as much as you might think. In our research, we have found virtually no difference in people's proneness to guilt (and no differences in shame either) as a function of religious background, at least when considering broad classes of religions represented in the United States (e.g., Catholic, Jewish, Protestant). We have examined this question across many different studies—those of children, college students, and parents and grandparents participating in our Longitudinal Family Study. Whether we considered current religious affiliation or religious affiliation in childhood, the results are pretty clear. No religion appears to have cornered the market on guilt.

Thus far, we have only considered broad categories of religion. It's possible that group differences may emerge from a more fine-grained analysis of religious beliefs and practices. For example, the degree of orthodoxy may be more important than broad differences in religious doctrine. Alternatively, the impact of religious background may hinge in part on one's ethnic or cultural background. The first author of this book, for example (a relatively shame-prone person), was raised in a Polish Catholic family that somehow gravitated to churches that emphasized human unworthiness and the threat of eternal suffering— churches that were populated with some of the most gruesome, bloody images from the Gospels. Her husband, on the other hand, was raised in an Irish Catholic family that emphasized Christian notions of agape, forgiveness, doing good, and helping others in the here and now. His Jesus was a kinder, gentler figure. His church featured symbols and images of hope and joy, not the blood and gore prevalent in some other parishes. He is not a shame-prone person.

In short, we can say with some confidence that American Catholics are not any more guilt-ridden (or shame-ridden) than their Protestant counterparts. Neither do people raised in a specific religion differ from those with no religious affiliation, in terms of "moral emotional style." Further research is needed, however, to take a more detailed look at the role of religion in the development of moral emotions.

Are There Gender Differences in the Propensity to Experience Shame and Guilt?

One of Freud's most controversial assertions is that women have a weaker, less internalized sense of morality than men, owing to defects in the formation of the superego. Freud (1923/1961d, 1924/1961c) suggested that because girls experience less castration anxiety during the Oedipal phase, the feminine superego is less solidly formed, resulting in an underdeveloped center of morality.

Given that shame and guilt are "superego" emotions, any gender difference in the strength or integrity of the superego should be directly observed in gender differences in feelings of shame and guilt. To what degree do men and women differ in their propensity to experience these moral emotions?

We have examined gender differences in proneness to shame and

guilt across our multiple studies totaling over 3,000 participants (Tangney & Dearing, in press). The consistency of results is striking.
Whether we considered elementary school-age children, lower middle-
class adolescents, college students, parents and grandparents of fifth-
grade students, or adult travelers passing through an airport, female
participants consistently report *greater* shame and guilt than their male
counterparts.[3]

In short, there is no evidence that women have defective superegos
as regards these quintessential superego emotions. At the same time, we
should note that these findings do not argue for moral superiority of
females either. As emphasized throughout this book, research indicates
that shame-proneness is the less adaptive moral emotional style, repeatedly linked to psychological symptoms (see Chapter 7), as well as such
"nonmoral" characteristics as an impaired capacity for other-oriented
empathy (Chapter 5). Compared to males, females across all ages report
a greater propensity to *both* shame and guilt. In this regard, girls and
women are the beneficiaries of the best and the worst of superego emotions.

Is There Any Evidence for a Genetic Basis for Moral Emotional Style?

In addition to socialization influences, biological factors may come into
play in the development of shame-proneness and guilt-proneness. To
our knowledge, only one study has directly examined the possibility of
a biological component in children's moral emotional style. In a study of
82 monozygotic and 78 dizygotic twins, Zahn-Waxler and Robinson
(1995) found a relatively strong genetic component for shame, with
correspondingly weak shared environment effects. For guilt, the opposite pattern was observed. Individual differences in guilt-proneness
appear more strongly tied to shared environment and less affected by
genetic factors.

Might there be certain key aspects of infant temperament that lay
the groundwork for shame-proneness or guilt-proneness? Developmental psychologists have identified a number of "temperament" dimensions that appear to be biologically based. Individual differences in temperament appear early in life and seem to be quite stable across the
lifespan. Dimensions of temperament that may be of special interest to
understanding the development of shame and guilt include fearfulness,
a propensity toward negative emotions in general, problems with self-

regulation, and shyness. One can imagine how a child who comes into the world with a biologically "hard-wired" fearfulness or sensitivity to negative emotions in general may be especially vulnerable to later tendencies toward shame and negative self-evaluation. Add to that biologically based difficulties with self-regulation and you may have a recipe for a shame-prone child.

Kochanska (1991, 1993) has developed a sophisticated model of early conscience development, suggesting that two dimensions of temperament, *affective discomfort* and *self-regulation,* interact with parental socialization practices. However, as mentioned previously, Kochanska does not distinguish between shame and guilt in her operationalization of "internalized conscience." Our guess is that temperamental fearfulness in a child, combined with parents who make frequent use of power-assertive, shame-inducing parenting practices, may be a potent combination for fostering the development of a shame-prone style. At the same time, this combination should be uniquely detrimental to the development of guilt. If such were the case, a blurring of shame and guilt would result in ambiguous findings because such differential relationships would essentially cancel one another out. Thus, a definitive test of these hypotheses remains a task for future research.

SUMMARY AND CONCLUSIONS

In this chapter, we focused on two questions related to the development of moral emotions. First, we looked at normative developmental changes in emerging shame and guilt. Across the lifespan, but especially in childhood, there are dramatic changes in self-concept, in the understanding and reasoning about moral issues, and in the degree to which shame and guilt are experienced as distinct emotions. Theory and some empirical evidence suggests that the capacity for shame emerges first— at about age 2. Guilt and the capacity to evaluate one's behavior independent of one's self almost certainly require a more sophisticated cognitive developmental level not typically seen much before age 8.

Normative developmental changes aside, there are substantial individual differences in moral emotional style. Our research has shown that, by at least middle childhood, people have a well-defined, consistent "moral emotional style." Some children are readily able to empathize with others; when they transgress, they are able to appropriately experience guilt, which then motivates them to take corrective action.

Other children, in contrast, show little sensitivity for the feelings of others; when they transgress, they may lack the capacity to feel a genuine sense of guilt or they may be inclined toward destructive feelings of shame which ultimately motivate denial, outwardly directed blame, and anger.

What individual, family, and other social factors help shape children's emerging tendencies to experience shame and guilt? Guilt-prone children perceive that their parents use behavior-focused messages and empathy induction when disciplining them. In contrast, shame-prone children report that their parents use person-focused disciplinary messages, express disgust, tease, communicate conditional approval, and use love-withdrawal techniques.

The ultimate value of understanding the factors that foster moral behavior lies in our ability to intervene. What can parents do to foster an "optimal" moral emotional style—for example, can we pinpoint specific disciplinary strategies that encourage an adaptive capacity for guilt versus maladaptive shame reactions? In Chapter 12, we take some beginning steps in this direction. Equally important, such information would help to identify young children "at risk" for maladaptive moral affective styles and patterns of behavior, and to develop appropriate early interventions.

NOTES

1. During the interviews conducted at age 18, index children were asked explicitly to identify their primary father figure. Where interview data were not available, we carefully examined the entire set of family data on a case-by-case basis.
2. The answer is "Yes" for Tangney and "No" for Dearing.
3. Note that our TOSCA measures are especially well suited to test Freud's assertions because of their scenario-based format. Some measures (e.g., the Revised Shame and Guilt Scale, the Personal Feelings Questionnaire) ask people how often they experience shame and guilt generally. The results using these general frequency measures would be somewhat equivocal because if women are indeed somehow morally inferior, they might engage in more frequent immoral acts on a day-to-day basis, and as a result, encounter more frequent opportunities to experience shame and guilt. Our TOSCA measures, on the other hand, present people with a standard set of gender-neutral situations. Thus, it is possible to examine gender differences in the likelihood of shame and guilt reactions with respect to the same set of events. Freud's theory clearly predicts lower levels of superego emotions (shame and guilt) among women than among men.

Chapter 10

SEX, ROMANCE, AND CONFLICT

Shame and Guilt
in Intimate Relationships

A man was walking along a California beach and stumbled across an old lamp. He picked it up and rubbed it and out popped a genie.

The genie said "OK, OK. You released me from the lamp, blah, blah, blah. This is the fourth time this month and I'm getting a little sick of these wishes so you can forget about three. You only get one wish!"

The man sat and thought about it for a while and said, "I've always wanted to go to Hawaii but I'm scared to fly and I get very seasick. Could you build me a bridge to Hawaii so I can drive over there to visit?"

The genie laughed and said, "That's impossible. Think of the logistics of that! It would have to be over a thousand miles long, with tens of thousands of supports, each over a mile long. Think of just how much concrete and steel that would require!! No, I can't do it, think of another wish."

The man said OK and tried to think of a really good wish.

Finally, he said, "I've never been able to please a woman—no matter how much I do for them, it's never enough. I wish that I could truly understand women . . . know what they really want . . . and know how to make them truly happy. . . . "

The genie's reply: "Do you want that bridge to be two lanes or four?"

—FROM JOKE FORWARDED VIA E-MAIL

As underscored by several recent bestsellers, men and women's contrasting communication styles often set the stage for misunderstandings. These misunderstandings are sometimes comical and sometimes heartbreaking and conflictual. Titles like J. Gray's *Men Are from Mars, Women Are from Venus* (1992) and D. Tannen's *You Just Don't Understand* (1990) convey the often vexing fundamental differences—at least as perceived by such popular authors and their reading public—between men and women in both their language and interpretation of events. In the clinical and research literature, too, these themes arise repeatedly, forming the basis for clinical interventions with distressed couples (Huber & Milstein, 1985; Rugel, 1997; Weiss & Halford, 1996). In reviewing this literature, we have been struck by how frequently unacknowledged shame appears to be the culprit in these miscommunications between couples.

Owing to their contrasting perspectives, couples may have particular difficulty communicating about their shame experiences. In describing couples' patterns of discussing personal "troubles," Tannen (1990) illustrates how partners' contrasting attempts to offer one another help ironically results in shaming each other further. Many, perhaps most, such personal troubles are shaming situations: worries about a job, a rift in an important relationship, sexual incompatibilities, concerns about health or physical attractiveness, and money are each potentially shame-inducing topics.

Although women may be more self-disclosing than men, in general, men and women *each* share woes and worries with their intimate partners. The problem is, they are apt to interpret their partner's needs in different ways (M. Lewis, 1992; Tannen, 1990). In offering help to their partners, women are inclined to express sympathy and share examples of their own similar experiences in an effort to convey the messages, "I understand you; you're not alone." In contrast, men are more likely to help by problem solving, offering suggestions, trying to come up with a solution and resolution. The woman is trying to nurture; the man is trying to repair. And both are caring responses! But often neither effort goes over very well.

As Tannen (1990) observes, women are apt to hear men's problem-solving efforts as unsympathetic, even belittling. What women want is a sympathetic ear; what they hear is an impatient, "Why don't you just fix it this way?"—often with the shaming message that they are incompetent (e.g., "Why didn't you fix it that way yourself in the first place?"). In turn, men are truly puzzled by their partners' lack of appreciation for their problem-solving efforts. Moreover, the rejection of their well-meaning offer of help is hurtful and, in many cases, shaming. The message is that they have failed in their role as protector; they are incompetent in those all-important problem-solving skills; they can't even come up with a useful (acceptable) suggestion.

It's not clear what exactly men are looking for when sharing their troubles, but what they typically get doesn't fit the bill. Because women find reassurance in expressions of empathy and sympathy, they are naturally moved to offer this form of help to their partners. But to everyone's dismay, women's offers of sympathy and empathic sharing of similar experiences are often not helpful. In fact, they can be experienced as downright shaming, trivializing the man's concerns and taking away his sense of uniqueness, according to Tannen (1990). In sharing their troubles, it's not clear that men want active problem solving either. Concrete practical suggestions can carry with them the metamessage that the man is incompetent, unable to cope on his own.

Rugel (1997), too, focuses on threats to self-esteem as a key component of conflict in romantic relationships, framing many of the difficulties experienced by marital partners in terms of gender differences in socialization. Men are socialized to develop an autonomous orientation—to strive for and value autonomy. Women, in contrast, are socialized to value and nurture relationships. Along similar lines, Helgeson (1994) contrasts the masculine "agency" orientation (focusing on self and separating from others) with the feminine "communal" orientation (focusing on others and forming connections). According to Rugel (1997), owing to this fundamental gender difference, men and women are vulnerable to self-esteem threats in different and sometimes conflicting domains. Most notably, women are inclined to interpret their partner's efforts at independence as a lack of connectedness, which in turn is often experienced as a devaluation of the relationship and a source of personal shame.

Tannen (1990) also emphasizes the special importance of status for men and interconnectedness for women. Whereas women are inclined to value and strive toward ideals of equality and community, men are sensitive to issues of status and rank. Drawing on physiological data from animal and human research, S. E. Taylor et al. (2000) provide strong empirical support for this fundamental gender difference, contrasting males' "fight-or-flight" orientation to females' characteristic "tend-and-befriend" responses to stress. In this light, it's interesting to consider two contrasting lines of theorizing about the "fundamental" roots of shame. Gilbert (1997; Gilbert & McGuire, 1998) and others (Keltner & Harker, 1998) focus on issues of rank, status, dominance, and submission—viewing shame as fundamentally linked to lowered status in social hierarchies. A second dominant theoretical account of the roots of shame focuses on threats to relationship bonds (H. B. Lewis, 1981, 1987a, 1987c; Scheff, 1997). From this perspective, shame is typically evoked by disrupted attachments, the experience of interpersonal loss or abandonment, and especially social rejection.

The stark contrast between these two theoretical accounts of shame is puzzling, but it may be better understood in light of Tannen's explanation of cross-gender miscommunication. Both accounts of shame would appear to have merit—one more characteristic of the experiences of men, and the other more characteristic of the experiences of women. In short, men are most often shamed by put-downs, rank issues, and other social status threats. Women are more often shamed by threats to attachment bonds.

A STUDY OF COUPLES IN CONFLICT: CONSTRUCTIVE VERSUS DESTRUCTIVE RESPONSES TO EVERYDAY ANGER

When people spend a lot of time together, especially when they live together, feelings of anger and conflict are inevitable. We can't help occasionally stepping on our partners' toes, engaging in irritating behavior, or making a thoughtless remark. One of the factors that undoubtedly contributes to a healthy relationship is the ability *not to avoid conflict* but to manage inevitable conflicts and disagreements in a constructive, proactive manner. This requires communication and understanding.

As part of a larger program of research on constructive versus destructive responses to anger, we studied romantically involved college-age couples as they grappled with the inevitable arguments and conflicts that arise in intimate relationships (Tangney, 2000). As discussed in greater detail in Chapter 6, participants (216 young adult couples) were interviewed in depth concerning specific real-life shared episodes of anger. Our couples described a broad range of anger-eliciting events. The factor we were particularly interested in was whether the offense caused the victim partner to feel shame. The couples' anger events were sorted into two categories: situations in which the angry victim was shamed, and situations in which the angry victim was not shamed. These "shame" and "non-shame" events were quite heterogeneous. In each case, they ranged from fairly trivial events (such as failing to show up for an appointment or date) to quite serious events (such as infidelity), and there was substantial overlap between the two lists (see Table 10.1). But shamed victims differed from nonshamed victims in the kinds of feelings they experienced; they differed in their intentions and responses toward the perpetrator; and they differed in their assessment of the long-term consequences of the event.

As described in greater detail in Chapter 6, victims of the shame-related anger events were significantly more angry, and more likely to report malevolent and fractious intentions (e.g., getting back at their partner, letting off steam) rather than trying to fix the situation. More importantly, shamed victims behaved differently from nonshamed victims in response to their anger. Relative to their nonshamed peers, shamed boyfriends reported more direct and indirect aggression—behaviors intended to cause harm to the perpetrating girlfriend. In contrast, shamed girlfriends were inclined toward displacing aggression onto someone or something other than their boyfriend. Shamed girlfriends were also apt to direct hostility inward, toward themselves. Not surprisingly, shamed victims felt bad about how they handled their anger. Shamed girlfriends were embarrassed, anxious, sad, shamed, and surprised. The aggressive shamed boyfriends felt dominant, sad, and ashamed.

It is notable that these apparently maladaptive expressions of anger did not result in any positive behavior on the part of the shame-inducing

---

TABLE 10.1. Examples of Couples' Anger-Eliciting Events

With victim shame

- He made a social engagement for the two of them without checking with her.
- She stood him up and went to lunch with another guy.
- He physically assaulted her during an argument.
- She didn't show up for dinner with his family.
- He was late meeting her after an exam.
- She dawdled and made them late for an appointment.
- He made negative comments about her mother.
- She complained and criticized his driving.

Without victim shame

- He didn't defend her when a friend blamed her for not inviting him to a party.
- She lied to him about having an affair.
- He promised to take her out but went out with his friends instead.
- She chewed with her mouth open during dinner.
- He insisted on picking up the car from the repair shop at an inconvenient time.
- She didn't get up on time to do a class assignment.
- He went out and drank excessively.
- She wasn't putting enough time and effort into the relationship.

perpetrators. Perpetrators were apt to respond to their shamed and aggressive partners with anger, resentment, defiance, and denial. They were less likely to respond with apologies and attempts to fix the situation, which were common responses among the nonshamed couples. In addition, couples' ratings of the long-term consequences of the anger episodes were more negative when anger was coupled with shame. Situations involving shamed boyfriends were rated as especially destructive, particularly from the girlfriends' perspective (which is not surprising, considering the shamed boyfriends' tendency toward overt aggression). The couples identified situations involving shamed girlfriends (who engaged in displaced and self-directed aggression) as less problematic.

In sum, findings regarding situation-specific feelings of shame in the midst of couples' real-life episodes of anger converge with results from dispositional studies linking trait shame with trait anger and maladaptive responses to anger (see Chapter 6). As shown in Figure 10.1, taken together, these data provide a powerful empirical example of the shame–rage spiral described by H. B. Lewis (1971) and Scheff (1987), with (1) victim shame leading to feelings of rage, (2) with destructive retaliation, (3) which then sets into motion partner anger and resentment, (4) as well as expressions of blame and retaliation in kind, (5) which is then likely to further shame the victim, and so forth—without any constructive resolution in sight.

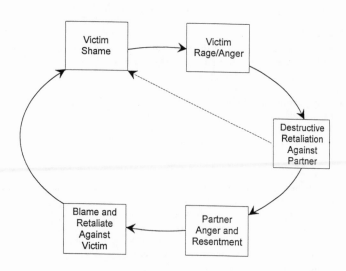

FIGURE 10.1. Shame and anger: From bad to worse.

THE SHAME-BOUND COUPLE

As highlighted in our study of a nonclinical sample of romantically involved college students, shame can wreak havoc in intimate relationships by setting in motion a cycle of escalating anger, externalization of
blame, and recurring shame. The prognosis for everyday conflicts
steeped in shame is grim. It should come as no surprise, then, that as
one looks at distressed relationships outside the norm, problems with
shame loom especially large.

In his discussion of domestic violence, Lansky (1987) has suggested that when two shame-prone individuals become romantically involved, the result is often disastrous. Not only do shame-prone partners
bring their own individual vulnerabilities to their relationship (e.g., insecure attachment, fear of negative evaluation, an impaired capacity for
empathy), but teamed up as a couple they are apt to form a "shame-
bound" system that only serves to exacerbate shame and conflict.
"Shame-bound" relationships are characterized by repeated rejection
and frequent messages of overt humiliation (Fossum & Mason; 1986;
Lansky, 1987) that do little to reassure partners of their self-worth or
the integrity of the relationship. Instead, the typical interaction just
rubs more salt on the wounds, capitalizing on and deepening the partner's vulnerability and sense of insecurity. This language of accusation,
blame, and humiliation contrasts sharply with the language of respect
characteristic of non-shame-bound relationships. Interactions in non-
shame-bound relationships foster a sense of security, cohesion, and
mutual care.

Another notable feature of shame-bound relationships is the need
to measure carefully, weigh, and assign blame. In the face of any negative outcome, large or small, *someone* or *something* must be found responsible (and held accountable). There's no notion of "water under
the bridge." Shame-prone couples are inclined to devote a great deal
of time and energy tossing back and forth the "hot potato" of blame.
After all, if *someone* must be to blame and it's not me, it must be you!

From blame comes shame. And then hurt, denial, anger, and retaliation. The irony here is that the types of defenses employed by shame-
prone partners ultimately do little to protect the self. Rather, such
chronic efforts at self-protection only serve to construct a relationship
that hits each partner where it hurts most, by escalating dramatically
the level of blame and shame (Lansky, 1987). For many distressed couples, it's an endless and self-perpetuating cycle.

TOWARD A RESOLUTION: APPRECIATING DIFFERENCES IN COMMUNICATION STYLES

Partners can reduce shame in their relationships by learning to recognize and respect differences in their concerns and in their patterns of communication. As partners develop an awareness of one another's unique perspective, they begin to minimize painful miscommunications and misunderstandings. As Tannen (1990) notes, "Many women could learn from men to accept some conflict and difference without seeing it as a threat to intimacy [or as a devaluation of the self], and many men could learn from women to accept interdependence without seeing it as a threat to their freedom" (p. 294).

An important benefit of recognizing differences in individual needs and communication style is that blame becomes a less prevalent feature of the relationship landscape. As Tannen (1990) further observed,

> Once people realize that their partners have different conversational styles, they're inclined to accept differences without blaming themselves, their partners, or their relationships. The biggest mistake is believing there is one right way to listen, to talk, to have a conversation—or a relationship. Nothing hurts more than being told your intentions are bad when you know they are good, or being told you are doing something wrong when you know you're just doing it your way. (pp. 297–298)

One hitch is that such perspective-taking requires a genuine sense of empathy, and (as discussed in Chapter 5) shame often interferes with people's ability to empathize. But practice helps!

THE ULTIMATE SHAME: ABUSE IN INTIMATE RELATIONSHIPS

At times, shame in intimate relationships can take a tragic, ugly turn. Domestic violence is a pervasive, heartbreaking problem in our society. In fact, intrafamilial violence is currently the most prevalent type of violent crime in the United States (Widom, 1989); 13% of all marriages involve chronic and severe violence (Straus, Gelles, & Steinmetz, 1980).

Not surprisingly, Dutton's (1998) research suggests that male batterers are, in fact, unusually shame-prone. And clinical accounts, too, underscore that problems with shame lie at the heart of abusive relationships (Dutton, 1995; Lansky, 1987). Dutton's (1998) clinical profile of the male batterer paints the picture of a jealous, insecure, easily threatened individual who attempts to cover his fear and shame with overt hostility and demands for control, especially within his most intimate—and therefore most dangerous—relationships.

Drawing from the works of P. Gilbert, D. Finkelhor, and others, B. Andrews (1998) makes a compelling case that the perpetrators of violence project their own "guilt and other bad feelings" (p. 181) onto their victims. Similarly, violent husbands often attempt to blame their abusive actions on the victim of the abuse, namely, their spouse (Holtzworth-Munroe & Hutchinson, 1993).

Victims of abuse are also likely to be shame-prone (Kessler & Bieschke, 1999) and, in turn, are likely to believe that they deserve to be treated poorly and are thus responsible for violent acts against them (B. Andrews, 1998). Thus, when blamed for the abuse by their violent husbands, these shame-prone women are likely to accept and internalize blame. By accepting this submissive role, victimized women may allow their abusive husbands to feel less shame (B. Andrews, 1998).

Dutton (1999) has suggested that the roots of spouse abuse run far into the early childhood experiences of batterers. There are indications that many men who abuse their partners were, as children, subjected to intense humiliation and shame by their parents (Dutton, 1995, 1998). In one study, for example, male batterers recalled a relatively high incidence of parental rejection and shaming, such as public scolding, "generic" criticism, and random punishment (Dutton, van Ginkel, & Starzomski, 1995). (See Chapter 12 for a discussion of shame-inducing and shame-reducing parenting strategies.) Further, physically violent men are likely to have been exposed to violent role models during childhood (Sugarman & Hotaling, 1989), suggesting a self-perpetuating cycle of domestic abuse.

SHAME IN THE BEDROOM: CAN THERE BE SEX WITHOUT SHAME?

John Bradshaw (1988) observed, "Perhaps no aspect of human activity has been as dysfunctionally shamed as much as our sexuality" (p. 54). From the get-go, children in our society are quickly taught, "Cover up! Don't look! Don't ask!" And *especially*, "Don't touch!"

In addition to these general prohibitions about sex, it is worth noting that men and women have some unique areas of vulnerability with regard to sexuality. For men, the big deal is *performance*. How big, how long, with whom, how many times, with what outcome? These are the dimensions of male evaluation—and represent their most likely Achilles' heel when it comes to shame in the bedroom. Men are vulnerable to feelings of shame for having too few "notches on the belt," for being "sized up" in the locker room (and coming up short), or for simply being "a sissy"—not assertive or masculine enough. Then there's the ultimate shame—the humiliating experience of impotence. (Even once in 20 years is enough to strike fear and insecurity in the heart of the most manly man.)

For women, the hot points for shame center on different issues. Women are faced with two conflicting sexual ideals—the chaste, pure, virginal bride in white versus the voluptuous, seductive, sex kitten. On the one hand, they are vulnerable to feelings of shame for being "too" sexual, having too many partners (loose women), or sending the wrong message (a tease). On the other hand, they are susceptible to feeling shame for being a prude, an ice queen, an old maid. In addition, the sex kitten ideal carries with it strong physical requirements—the "perfect 10." More generally, women are bombarded with unrealistic physical images of the feminine ideal—from Barbie to Supermodel. It's clearly a no-win situation.

Men and women may start out with different sources of shame about sex, but when they get together in the bedroom one partner's shame often triggers shame in the other. M. Lewis (1992) commented on the contagious nature of shame, particularly in the sexual arena. Consider, for example, one man's story of not feeling understood by his partner. Bob suffers from impotence due to medication he is currently taking. His partner, Sally, insists that his lack of arousal is a reflection of her physical appearance—she thinks that she's overweight and less than attractive to Bob. Sally "knows" that impotence is one of the common side effects of Bob's medication. But despite Bob's repeated explanations, Sally's focus remains on her own area of vulnerability—her physical appearance. In her heart, she's unable to attribute Bob's sexual difficulties to his medical condition. As a result, Bob feels misunderstood, brushed aside, and shamed by his inability to perform sexually, but now he is further distressed by his inability to help Sally feel adequate and reassured.

SHAME AND THE SEXUAL MINORITY

Human sexuality spans a broad spectrum (Freud coined the term "polymorphous perversity" to describe the diversity and plasticity of human sexuality), only part of which is considered socially acceptable or "normal" within a given culture. Cultures may vary in what is considered acceptable, and certain segments may be more or less accepting of sexual diversity. The critical point here is that within every society substantial aspects of human sexuality are considered deviant—and therefore *shameful*.

Being sexually different—belonging to a sexual minority—is a virtual guarantee of being socially rejected and stigmatized in many circles. Homosexuality is perhaps the most obvious example. Scientists estimate that roughly 5% of the population identify themselves as homosexual or bisexual (Diamond, 1993; Seidman & Rieder, 1994). As Kaufman and Raphael (1997) observe, this sexual minority has been stigmatized throughout the ages: "Homosexuality has been variously conceived and characterized as immorality, as against nature, as gender disturbance, and as mental illness" (p. 77). The stigmatization of homosexuality begins early in childhood and intensifies during adolescence, when slurs such as "queer," "faggot," "lesbo," and "dyke" are commonly used to ridicule and shame peers. Long before children begin to grapple with their own sexual orientation, they learn quite clearly that it is shameful to be "gay." It is no surprise, then, that many gay and lesbian adolescents stay locked "in the closet." And this secrecy, in turn, only serves to intensify a deep-rooted sense of shame. As Kaufman and Raphael (1997) note, "Silence breeds shame every bit as much as shame breeds further silence" (p. 103).

From this perspective, one can understand the sense of relief and emerging pride that often results from "coming out"—even when revelations about one's sexual orientation are not uniformly greeted with acceptance. Again, Kaufman and Raphael (1997) observe, "By coming out of the closet . . . we are coming out of shame, out of hiding, and coming not only into openness but into our own" (p. 105).

One tragic irony of the stigmatization of minorities—sexual or otherwise—is that shameful oppression does not always breed empathy for members of other stigmatized or marginalized groups. In many cases, feelings of shame and humiliation seem to drive members of one "outgroup" to recapture a sense of legitimacy and power by shaming and rejecting another—a "minority group within the minority group." As one poignant example of this self-perpetuating cycle of ostracism and shame, Riki Wilchins (1997) chronicles her life as a transsexual, describing in excruciating detail the pain and humiliation of being rejected by the lesbian "establishment." She relates her experiences at the much-anticipated Michigan Womyn's Music Festival, when organizers of the festival publicly excluded transgender "freaks," limiting the event to "womyn-born womyn only."

VENEREAL SHAME AND SEXUALLY TRANSMITTED DISEASES

Sexually transmitted diseases (STDs) may be a quintessential source of shame. STDs bring together shame and stigma from several sources. Our almost innate vulnerability to shame about sex is further compounded by the stigma of disease and then made even more profound by concerns of being judged as sinful, morally depraved, or irresponsible. To make matters worse, to obtain treatment for their condition, individuals suffering from STDs must make their condition public, at least in the sense of consulting with a medical practitioner. As patients, they must disclose and discuss private details about their sexual history and practices. It's no wonder that many people infected with STDs avoid or unduly postpone seeking medical help. In fact, a study of sexually active adults who suspected they had a STD reported that 27% delayed seeking treatment for at least 4 weeks (Leenaars, Rombouts, & Kok, 1993). In this context, too, shame no doubt motivates avoidance, escape, and denial.

Feelings of shame may not only deter people from seeking treatment. Even for those who seek medical treatment, feelings of shame can interfere with patients' acquisition of health-related knowledge and their motivation to comply with the recommended treatment regimen. For example, in a recent study of 205 adults living with HIV, Borenstein and Tangney (2001) found that HIV-related shame was inversely related to health-related knowledge, which in turn resulted in fewer health-related behaviors, thus compromising patients' long-term health. These results suggest that treatment of STDs may be substantially enhanced by an awareness of and sensitivity to patients' feelings of shame.

One of the most difficult dilemmas facing individuals infected with STDs is whether, how, and when to broach the topic with current and prospective sexual partners. For example, in one study, 20% of male college students reported that they would lie to a prospective sexual partner, claiming to have had a negative HIV test (Cochran & Mays, 1990). Even more alarming, 52% of sexually active HIV-positive males studied by Marks, Richardson, and Maldonado (1991) neglected to disclose their HIV status to sexual partners. Although there is as yet no systematic research on the topic, it seems likely that feelings of shame lie close to the heart of people's reluctance to responsibly inform partners and to take appropriate precautions.

Anecdotal evidence suggests that sometimes there's a strong element of anger and hostility in people's failure to inform partners about their disease status. For example, Shilts's (1987) historical chronicle of the AIDS virus describes in detail the pivotal role played by Gaetan Dugas in disseminating the epidemic in the United States. For years, Dugas purposely engaged in unprotected sex with literally hundreds of partners, even when repeatedly warned by physicians that he was most likely spreading the deadly disease. A man who had long prided himself on his striking good looks and attractiveness, Dugas felt considerable shame over the disfiguring lesions characteristic of Kaposi's sarcoma and a seething rage that someone had "done this" to him. Dugas struck back with a vengeance by frequenting gay bathhouses across the country. After anonymous sex in a darkened room, he was reported to turn up the lights and point out his Kaposi's sarcoma lesions, saying, "I've got gay cancer . . . I'm going to die and so are you" (p. 165). The consequences of Dugas's shame and anger were disastrous. Of the first 248 gay men in the world who were diagnosed with AIDS, at least 40 had sex either with Dugas or with someone sexually linked with him. The epidemic has since spread to millions worldwide.

In such instances, feelings of anger rather than shame appear most prominent. It's our strong guess, however, that such anger and hostility originates in the infected individual's sense of shame, humiliation, and powerlessness. As discussed at greater length in Chapter 6, feelings of shame not infrequently motivate a desire to strike back or lash out at others.

Of course, shame-induced anger is not limited to potential sexual partners. People suffering from STDs, especially chronic conditions such as AIDS, may be inclined to vent their anger on those involved in their care—medical staff, hospice workers, and significant others—pushing away much needed care and support. In this context, as in so many others, shame drives people apart when they need each other most.

SUMMARY AND CONCLUSIONS

Communication and understanding are essential components of any relationship, but they are especially crucial in our most intimate relationships. This chapter examined the many ways in which shame can crop up in our closest relationships—as both a cause and a result of miscommunication and misunderstanding. Owing to their different emphasis on status versus connection, men and women view their joint worlds from quite distinct perspectives. Thus, at times partners inevitably misconstrue one another's messages and intentions. These misunderstandings can result in hurt feelings, animosity, and—not infrequently—shame. Shame pulls people apart and damages connections. But partners can do much to minimize painful miscommunications and misunderstandings by developing an awareness of one another's unique perspective. Further, by recognizing and respecting differences, blame becomes less prevalent in the relationship.

Without question, sex is a "hotbed" of shame in our society. This is another area where tolerance and perspective taking can play an important role in enhancing intimacy and minimizing shame. In the domain of sex, shame exerts some of its most tragic consequences—wrenching apart loving relationships, marginalizing individuals in "sexual minorities," and fueling the spread of AIDS and other STDs. At its worst, shame inhibits safe sex practices, which require cooperation and open communication, while also discouraging infected individuals from seeking prompt and appropriate treatment. Perspective taking, tolerance for our inevitable differences, and sensitivity to experiences of shame (in ourselves and our partners) can go a long way toward strengthening our intimate bonds—and saving lives.

Chapter 11

IMPLICATIONS FOR THERAPISTS

Shame and Guilt on
Both Sides of the Couch

The context of psychotherapy lends itself to the consideration of shame from many different angles. As we have discussed in previous chapters, shame has a myriad of negative implications, ranging from strained interpersonal relations to a strong link with many types of psychological symptoms. Thus, a consideration of shame-related issues may be useful on several levels in the context of therapy. In particular, therapists may enhance their effectiveness with clients by keeping in mind the subtle but critical distinction between shame and guilt.

In this chapter, we discuss therapy as a context that lends itself to problematic feelings of shame on multiple levels. Shame is ubiquitous in the problems that lead clients into therapy, and for better or worse it is part of the therapeutic process itself. We describe verbal and nonverbal indicators of underlying shame reactions, and suggest therapeutic strategies to help clients cope with shame. We also note that issues of shame stretch beyond the client–therapist interaction, affecting family members and significant others of those suffering from psychological disorders. Finally, therapists are not immune to reactions of shame themselves. We discuss some of the special shame-related issues that arise owing to the therapist's professional role.

THERAPY: A CONTEXT FRAUGHT
WITH EXPERIENCES OF SHAME

In our society, there is an undeniable stigma associated with being a patient with psychological problems. People who seek psychological help have essentially identified themselves as deficient, defective, and in need of repair. And they are likely to assume that others will see them this way as well—faulty, weak, and unable to cope with life on their own. Not surprisingly, a common fear of therapy clients is that others will find out about their problems and/or patient status. Many prospective clients fear the shame of being identified as a "mental patient."

Not surprisingly, many people who could benefit from psychological treatment never make it into therapy. Based on a review of the psychological help-seeking literature, Kushner and Sher (1991) concluded that only about 20% of individuals with a significant mental disorder seek help. Numerous "barriers"—real and perceived—impede distressed individuals from seeking treatment (Fee, 1998). For example, in a study of college students, 51% indicated that the anticipation of shame was at least "moderately important" in their decision of whether to enter therapy. Moreover, shame-prone individuals perceived greater barriers to seeking help.

For those who finally overcome such barriers to seeking help, what awaits them are a host of potentially shaming interactions during treatment. Psychotherapy is a process that by its very nature involves an acute focus on self, especially the feared, problematic aspects of self. Clients are encouraged to reveal their deepest, darkest, most painful secrets—their otherwise carefully concealed flaws. To make matters worse, these painful, shame-inducing revelations are made before a therapist assumed to be a paragon of mental health. From the perspective of many clients, this is a shameful comparison—a needy, fragile, incompetent, "ill" client meets the all-knowing, healthy, wise therapist!

Not only is the *reality* of the therapeutic context likely to induce feelings of shame, but clients' experiences in therapy are often complicated by the process of "transference," whereby patients "transfer" the perceptions and dynamics of previous relationships onto their relationship with the therapist (Stadter, 1996; I. B. Weiner, 1998). Moreover, as clinicians are well aware, such "therapeutic transferences" are not typically derived from the most positive relationships in the client's past. In fact, there's good reason to suspect that clients differentially select and project shame-based relationship issues onto the client–therapist relationship. In their quest for help, clients are inclined to bring more shame into an already shame-laden situation.

In short, the context of psychotherapy is by its nature a shame-inducing relationship aimed at exploring shameful issues. Ironically, the very people who are most likely to enter therapy are shame-prone people. As discussed in Chapter 7, people prone to the ugly feeling of shame are vulnerable to a range of psychological symptoms. It follows, then, that many of the clients seeking therapy for psychological problems are predisposed to the experience of shame to begin with.

HOW SHAME COMPLICATES
THE THERAPEUTIC PROCESS

We have discussed numerous ways in which the process of therapy can elicit shame. What is the impact of such experiences of shame on the treatment process and its outcome? Throughout the preceding chapters, we have emphasized the painful nature of shame and the difficulties people have in resolving this aversive emotion. We have discussed at length how the pain of shame can lead either to withdrawal from interpersonal interactions or to a hostile humiliated fury. Shame-induced withdrawal and/or anger can be readily observed in the context of psychotherapy as well.

A common component of the shame experience is the desire to hide, to escape from further scrutiny and devaluation. In effect, the shamed self seeks to "sink into the floor and disappear." We shouldn't be surprised to see this reaction in the therapy room, too. Movement toward withdrawal, concealment, and escape can be manifest in numerous client behaviors, many of which fall under the general heading of "resistance." Psychotherapists have long recognized that, somewhat paradoxically, clients can be their own worst enemy when it comes to effective treatment (Cashdan, 1988; I. B. Weiner, 1998). That is, it's not uncommon for psychotherapy patients to interfere with, interrupt, or in some other way directly undermine the very process on which progress hinges. In fact, therapeutic resistance is such a widely recognized phenomenon in treatment that clinicians are taught that client resistance can be a "red flag" that the therapy has stumbled onto a "hot" but repressed client issue (Stadter, 1996).

Resistance in the therapy session can also serve as a red flag that the client is experiencing shame. Although shame is a common emotion (especially in the therapeutic process), people rarely announce that they are feeling shame (H. B. Lewis, 1971). In fact, shame is one of the most frequently overlooked emotions—by the person experiencing shame, as well as by others in the immediate social context. When a client arrives late for a session, misses an appointment, abruptly changes the subject, or claims to have "nothing to say," shame may very well be the source of the problem.

As described in Chapter 6, research has shown that shame not only motivates a desire to hide, escape, or avoid shame-eliciting situations but can also provoke feelings of rage and anger. Often, such shame-based anger is not a rational response, warranted by the facts of the situation. On even the flimsiest grounds, shamed individuals may be drawn to direct the blame outward, to become angry in an attempt to rescue themselves from threatening, distressing feelings of shame. In the context of therapy, such shame-to-anger transformations might be seen in a variety of negative transference reactions—anger and resentment toward the therapist being the most common. For example, clients may become irritated and blame the therapist for misunderstandings about clearly stated appointment times, payment/insurance issues, and the like. They may berate the therapist for simply "not caring enough." They may contentiously question the therapist's skills, abilities, or credentials. Or they may experience rage toward the therapist for being "made" to feel so bad. In short, shamed clients may become unaccountably argumentative, belligerent, or otherwise hostile in the midst of an apparently productive session.

Thus, when the flow of the therapeutic interaction grinds to a halt, when the client responds to the therapist with seemingly irrational anger, or when the client suddenly and inexplicably decides to end treatment, the possibility of an underlying sense of shame vis-à-vis the therapist might be considered.

HOW CAN THERAPISTS RECOGNIZE EXPERIENCES OF SHAME?

One problem posed by shame is that clients typically have difficulty identifying and verbalizing the shame experience. Helen Block Lewis (1971) noted the primitive, nonverbal nature of shame, based on her clinical case studies. This inability to identify and articulate episodes of shame may, in part, account for the persistent nature of the shame experience. And this characteristic may also cause therapists to overlook significant shame episodes experienced by their clients.

In treating clients, it is helpful to listen with a "third ear" for shame-based experiences. Clients often provide subtle cues that signal the possibility of a shame episode. There may be an abrupt interruption in a client's account of previous events, accompanied by signs of discomfort or agitation, nervous laughter, and/or downcast eyes. Other potential clues to an underlying shame reaction include gaze aversion, face touching, lip manipulation, and a slumped posture (Covert, 2000; Keltner, 1995; Keltner & Buswell, 1996; M. Lewis, 1992). In addition, the client may have difficulty articulating his or her experience of the moment. On the other hand, as discussed above, clients may provide more overt evidence of a shame reaction in the form of disproportionate expressions of anger.

HELPING CLIENTS COPE WITH SHAME

What sorts of interventions are effective in diffusing shame reactions?

First, simply verbalizing the events and associated experiences often serves to ameliorate the feeling of shame. As clients translate into words their preverbal, global shame reaction, they bring to bear a more logical, differentiated thought process that may compel them to spontaneously reevaluate the global nature of the shame-eliciting episode. For example, a client may experience unacknowledged shame for changing a scheduled appointment due to a family emergency. The alert therapist, noting the client's shift in affect coupled with subtle nonverbal signs, might help the client recognize the underlying sense of shame. As the client verbalizes this shame, she may realize, upon further examination, that the event was truly beyond her control and that there was simply no cause for shame—disappointment and frustration, maybe, but not shame. Had the therapist not picked up on these subtle cues, that irrational sense of shame might have persisted throughout the session, wreaking havoc with subsequent attempts to address salient client concerns already on the table.

Second, in the process of exploring the shame-eliciting episode, the therapist can further assist the client in making such cognitive reevaluations. In fact, many of the key cognitive-behavioral interventions for depression described by Beck (1983) and Ellis (1962) are likely to be an effective means of addressing shame-inducing cognitions. Shame, too, is associated with irrational beliefs and dysfunctional thoughts that are amenable to cognitive restructuring. Therapists can take an active role in helping clients step back and look at "the forest instead of the trees." Many clients benefit from explicit efforts to put specific failures, shortcomings, or misdeeds in the larger context of their habits, abilities, and life experiences. It's a fact that most flaws, setbacks, and oversights really *don't* warrant global feelings of worthlessness or shame.

Third, therapists can encourage such "contextualization" by explicitly educating the client about the difference between shame and guilt. A surprising observation from our clinical work is that many clients really have not considered the difference between condemning a behavior and condemning the self. Given an explicit choice, many spontaneously shift the focus of negative judgments from the global self to a specific behavior. They simply do not realize that behavior-focused feelings of guilt are an option. Therapists can further encourage clients to make a conscious shift from a shame-prone style to a guilt-prone style by discussing and reinforcing an appreciation of the problematic aspects of shame versus the potentially adaptive functions of guilt.

Fourth, in sharing shame experiences within the context of a supportive relationship, clients typically meet with acceptance and understanding. In discussing the fundamental elements of successful psychotherapy, Rogers (1975) emphasized the importance of communicating "unconditional positive regard" toward the client. Therapists may not positively regard or condone every action of a client, but therapists *can* provide a warm accepting climate for the client as a person. In a similar vein, Linehan (1993a, 1993b) has emphasized the importance of helping clients accept themselves as they are in the moment, while also acknowledging the need and desire for change. An important component of the therapist's role is to help clients value themselves as individuals, independent of their presenting psychopathology. The upshot is that as clients reveal their secret shame-eliciting fears, flaws, and foibles over the course of treatment, the therapist's reaction provides clients with an alternative to the self-disgust and self-disdain inherent in the shame experience.

Finally, Retzinger (1987) has presented data suggesting that humor may be an effective antidote to shame. Light-hearted humor, by its very nature, normalizes individual shortcomings, thus placing them in a more realistic perspective. There's much to be said for the notion that "laughter is the best medicine." The levity inherent in playful humor is incompatible with the harsh, deadly serious self-condemnation of shame. As clients bring dreaded shame experiences to light, a shared joke about some irony of the situation, or about the disproportionate nature of their shame reaction, can help dispel the ugly feeling of shame. Here, it is critical for clients to experience the therapist as laughing *with*—not *at*—them. There is often a fine line between a friendly, inclusive, humorous joke and a hurtful, mocking putdown (Gessner & Tangney, 1990).

Shame Reaching Beyond the Therapy Room: Family Members and Involved Others

Although often overlooked, clients' friends and family members may also be vulnerable to experiences of shame. Friends and family members of distressed clients seeking therapy may wonder how they may have contributed to their loved one's problems. They may take their loved one's need for professional help as a sign of failure in their role as parent, spouse, or close confidant. Or they may wonder if others are assuming that they must be bad parents (or bad spouses, children, or siblings).

Significant others may also worry that, in the course of treatment, the client will disclose intimate details about their relationship in a way that would reflect negatively on them, particularly given that they won't be present to defend themselves. In fact, friends or family members actively may discourage clients from seeking treatment, anticipating shame at the prospect of having their own "dirty laundry" revealed to the therapist. Further, there may be shame simply in being closely associated with someone who is experiencing "psychological problems," owing to the stigma attached to mental illness in our culture (Wahl, 1995).

SHAME AMONG COUNSELORS AND THERAPISTS

Shame is not a one-way street in the emotionally charged therapy room. Therapists, too, are vulnerable to painful, sometimes overwhelming experiences of shame. Most therapists' identities center on being a warm, empathic, wise, and effective helping professional. It's the nature of the job that this identity is challenged on a day-to-day basis. On a bad day, a therapist may confront multiple shaming experiences—from one client after another.

Numerous sources of shame confront therapists. As discussed earlier, clients themselves inevitably experience shame in the course of treatment. Shamed clients are inclined to lash out at therapists in a variety of ways that can be shame-inducing—for example, questioning the therapist's skills, abilities, or credentials; blaming the therapist for lack of progress; accusing the therapist of "not really understanding"; or leaving therapy altogether. Therapists are human beings, each with his or her own limitations. It goes without saying that the "helper" may, from time to time, feel shame and/or anger in response to such affronts. Owing to their professional role and related self-expectations, therapists may further feel ashamed for simply reacting with feelings of shame, anger, and resentment toward the client whom they are supposedly to help—with unconditional positive regard, even.

Clients themselves are not the only source of therapists' shame. Clinicians have long noted that "countertransference" reactions are an inevitable component of the therapeutic process. In countertransference, the therapist's reaction to a client is colored by his or her own personal dynamics and past relationships (I. B. Weiner, 1998). In effect, these personal therapist issues are unconsciously "transferred" onto the relationship with the client. Countertransference reactions can be both positive and negative in valence, and each poses special challenges to the alert clinician. In a negative countertransference reaction, the therapist—often inexplicably—develops negative attitudes and reactions toward the client and his or her therapy. The therapist may feel annoyed, bored, disgusted, impatient, or downright angry with the client. And such reactions often seem out of proportion to the facts of the interaction, in retrospect.

Negative countertransference reactions can be especially insidious to the therapeutic relationship, and it is our guess that unrecognized bouts of shame are a critical component of many negative countertransference reactions. Negative countertransference can be provoked when clients inadvertently activate the therapist's own shameful fears and insecurities. On the flip side, therapists are apt to feel shame simply because they harbor ill will toward the client—an experience so at odds with their role as a warm, accepting, empathic helping professional. To make matters worse, we know from our research that shame often motivates a desire to withdraw, deny, or externalize blame. Thus, the therapist's first natural reaction under such circumstances may be to deny these negative feelings, blame the client, or withdraw (emotionally or physically) from the therapeutic process. Effective therapists are alert to the possibility of countertransference, and their effectiveness may be enhanced to the extent that they can recognize and work through associated feelings of shame.

Finally, therapists are vulnerable to feelings of shame in the face of therapeutic failure. As trained helping professionals, therapists inevitably have a vested interest in the outcome of treatment. The skill of the therapist is assumed to be reflected in client progress and improvement. When the work goes well, we congratulate ourselves for our clinical acumen. When things go poorly, we blame ourselves. Unfortunately, therapy failures are not uncommon. Some therapies—especially those involving Axis II diagnoses—go on for months, even years, with little sign of improvement. Some clients terminate prematurely. Some clients experience unanticipated crises, setbacks, and/or hospitalization. And then there is the ultimate failure—a client's suicide. Estimates of the percentage of therapists who have lost a patient to suicide range from 15-51% (Brown, 1987; Chemtob, Hamada, Bauer, Kinney, & Torigoe, 1988; Kahne, 1968; Litman, 1965). Common reactions to therapy failures include anger, shock, denial, anxiety, shame and embarrassment, as well as a loss of confidence and self esteem (Chemtob et al., 1988; Meade, personal communication, 1998). In fact, Chemtob et al. (1988) found that shortly after patients' suicides, psychiatrists reported stress levels that were comparable to those of individuals seeking therapy after the death of a parent.

SUMMARY AND CONCLUSIONS

Feelings of shame are an inevitable and integral part of the psychotherapeutic process. First, as discussed in Chapter 7, shame-prone individuals are more vulnerable to psychological problems and thus are more likely to be in need of psychological treatment. Second, the nature of the therapeutic process itself is often shame eliciting. In the context of therapy, clients are expected to reveal painful failures and shortcomings that can cause shame. Third, feelings of shame—whether on the part of the client or the therapist—can interfere with the progress of therapy. One important characteristic of effective and resilient therapists may be their ability to identify and resolve shameful feelings constructively. Similarly, a key component of successful psychotherapy is helping clients develop skills to weather the unavoidable experiences of shame in daily life.

Chapter 12

LOOKING AHEAD

*Implications for Parents,
Teachers, and Society*

The major "take-home" message from our book is that, over the years, guilt has received a bad rap. In a rush to free ourselves from a repressive, "old-fashioned" morality, we may have dismissed too quickly the adaptive functions of guilt. In the course of day-to-day life, people *do* occasionally transgress, offend, or otherwise cause harm to others. It may be uncomfortable but still adaptive (for ourselves and others) to experience guilt in connection with such specific behavioral transgressions. The tension, remorse, and regret of guilt causes us to stop and re-think—and it offers a way out, pressing us to confess, apologize, and make amends. We become better people, and the world becomes a better place.

In contrast, shame appears to be the less "moral" emotion in several important regards. When people feel ashamed of themselves, they are not particularly motivated to apologize and attempt to repair the situation. This is *not* an emotion that leads people to responsibly own up to their failures, mistakes, or transgressions and make things right. Instead, they are inclined to engage in all sorts of defensive maneuvers. They may withdraw and avoid the people around them. They may deny responsibility and blame others for the shame-eliciting situation. They may become downright hostile and angry at a world that has made them feel so small. In short, shamed individuals are inclined to assume a defensive posture, rather than take a constructive, reparative stance in their relationships.

From society's perspective, it may be helpful under very rare and extreme circumstances to have a mechanism that encourages "shameful" people (e.g., habitual rapists, child molesters, serial killers) to remove themselves from the social milieu. But, for the average person, shame is an inordinately harsh penalty for the inevitable failures and transgressions of daily life.

IMPLICATIONS FOR PARENTS: RAISING A MORAL CHILD

One of the most important parts of the job of parents is to teach their children to be good, moral, caring people. Most parents want their children to develop into adults who are sensitive and responsive to other people's feelings and needs. An important component of this process is to instill in children a clear sense of right and wrong, the ability to recognize when they transgress, and the motivation to do something about it. In short, parents aim to help their children develop into responsible members of society, with an awareness of and concern for their effect on others.

At the same time, no one wants to raise constricted, self-punitive, neurotic children—children who are petrified of making mistakes and far too quick to blame themselves for the woes of the world. Ideally, one would hope for moral *and* happy, emotionally well-adjusted children who have a solid and enduring sense of self-esteem.

How can parents best accomplish these two sometimes conflicting tasks? Parents really face a fundamental paradox. On the one hand, parents are the primary source of love and nurturance during a child's formative years. There is no greater love and attachment than that of a parent. Parents naturally want to give their children all the best that the world has to offer. A fundamental parenting goal is to promote children's feelings of security, happiness, and joy, and to shield them from pain and distress. On the other hand, parents also serve as the child's primary disciplinary figures. In this role, parents take primary responsibility for teaching their child the difference between right and wrong, and making them feel bad when they do bad things. And here's where the paradox comes in: On a regular basis, loving responsible parents must actually induce their children to feel bad. The typical parent engages in countless disciplinary actions in the course of an ordinary day.

This paradox poses an often unrecognized dilemma for loving parents. Making children feel bad seems at odds with most parents' attempts to provide an ideal world for their children. Moreover, parents' decisions about appropriate punishment are likely to be complicated by their own emotional reaction to their children's misbehavior. No parent is immune to the very human emotions of anger, resentment, exasperation, and disappointment. Children are expert at eliciting these and many other emotions on a day-to-day basis. Parental anger and resentment are likely, precisely at the very time when they are called upon to assume the role of disciplinarian. As a result, parents may feel guilty or ashamed of inflicting punishment and inducing the child's ensuing distress. For many parents, it is difficult to tease out their motivations for punishment: Is the nature of the disciplinary action guided by parental anger or by concern for the welfare of the child? In processing their reaction to the event, parents may question whether they are really trying to correct the child's behavior or just trying to make the child feel bad. In questioning their motives, parents may be inclined to blame themselves for acting out of anger, because the alternative—concern for the welfare of the child—seems at odds with punishing and inducing distress.

But concern for the welfare of a child is *not* at odds with discipline-induced distress, to the extent that the parent keeps in mind that there are good and bad ways to feel bad. Throughout this book, we have emphasized the adaptive functions of guilt in contrast to the costs of shame. A great deal of accumulated research indicates that guilt is a constructive, future-oriented, moral emotion that enhances our relationships with others. Thus, parents can do their children a service by teaching them to feel bad about bad behaviors but *not* bad about themselves. In this way, parents guide their children to be moral, responsible, happy, and well adjusted.

Key Components of Successful Parenting

Developmental psychologists have identified several elements that form the foundation of effective, healthy discipline (Baumrind, 1967, 1971; Dix, 1991; Grusec & Goodnow, 1994). First, children benefit from clear standards and expectations. Children are raised, not born, to be moral beings, and as such they need to be taught right from wrong (Dekovic & Janssens, 1992). Thus, parents must clearly communicate their values, expectations, and rules of conduct. Children need to know what is right in order to act appropriately.

Consistency is an important element of effective discipline (Maccobby & Martin, 1983; Patterson, 1982). Children need consistent feedback regarding the consequences of their actions. Young children and adolescents alike are apt to become confused, for example, if they are disciplined for hitting a sibling one day but let off the hook for doing the same thing the next day. Along the same lines, children benefit when both parents are in regular agreement regarding family rules and disciplinary strategies (Block, Block, & Morrison, 1981; Christensen, Margolin, & Sullaway, 1992). Further, parents and teachers are each likely to be more successful to the extent that they can support rather than undermine each other's standards and expectations.

Children are most likely to thrive in a loving and nurturing environment. They are more apt to learn from parental discipline when it's delivered in the context of a warm, loving relationship (Dix, 1991; Gottman & Declaire, 1998; Hoffman, 1970; Yarrow, Waxler, & Scott, 1971). Children who love and respect their parents—and feel love and respect in return—are more likely to embrace their parents' values and standards. They are less likely to discount or reject parental guidance and feedback.

In matters of discipline, more is not necessarily better. From our perspective, discipline is most effective when the focus is on "rehabilitation" as opposed to punishment. That is, the ultimate aim is not to cause pain, to retaliate, or to "punish for punishment's sake." Rather, the goal is use negative consequences to make children *notice* that they have transgressed, to *reflect* on their behavior and its consequences, and to make *positive changes* for the future. This use of punishment in service of repair is likely to be enhanced when discipline is matched to the nature and severity of the infraction.

Children need to know *what to do* as well as *what not to do*. It may be obvious to a parent that a child should ask for a turn at the Nintendo game, rather than grabbing the paddle from his or her sibling. But children, especially young children, are limited in their ability to generate alternative solutions in the heat of the moment. Child development experts emphasize the importance of using "positive" disciplinary messages whenever possible, guiding children *toward* desired behavior, rather than *away* from undesirable actions (Lytton, 1980; Belsky, Woodworth, & Crnic, 1996).

Successful discipline hinges on parents gearing their expectations and punishments to their child's developmental level (Kuczynski, Kochanska, Radke-Yarrow, & Girnius-Brown, 1987; Maccoby & Martin, 1983). Well-meaning parents sometimes set themselves (and their children) up for failure by expecting the impossible. For example, one can reasonably expect an 8-year-old to resist the temptation of a newly baked cake set out on the table to cool. A 2-year-old simply hasn't developed the self control to refrain from diving in while Mom's on the phone. One key to success is realistic expectations and developmentally appropriate punishment.

A Guilt-Inducing, Shame-Reducing Approach to Parenting

Whatever the child's developmental level, in the long run guilt-inducing discipline is likely to be more effective than shaming tactics. What parental behaviors are likely to result in a guilt-inducing, shame-reducing style of discipline? At present, there is little direct research to guide us on this issue; however, K. L. Rosenberg (1998) has shown that children's moral emotional style is linked strongly to their perceptions of parental discipline. And these findings converge with good common sense, as well as with the child development literature. How can parents best teach their children to respond adaptively to their inevitable failures and transgressions?

1. *Accentuate the behavior, not the person.* When disciplining children, it's easy to make the mistake of focusing on who they are, as people, rather than what they have *done* wrong. Adaptive feelings of guilt are more likely to result from behavior-focused here-and-now statements such as "John, you *did* a bad thing there when you . . . " as opposed to "John, you're a bad [mean, clumsy] *boy,*" or, more subtly "John, you're so *stupid* [careless, lazy, etc.]."

2. *Focus on the consequences for others.* As discussed in Chapter 5, empathy and guilt go hand in hand. Thus, it's important to help children recognize the effect of their behavior on others. Compared to adults, children tend to be self-centered and are less inclined to notice their impact on others. This is developmentally normal—the more so, the younger the child. So it can be very helpful to shift the child's attention with statements such as "Mary, it's not OK to hit Susie like that. Look at how that hurts Susie. She's crying." In this way, parents simultaneously focus the child's attention on the bad behavior (not his or her bad self) and on the consequences for others.

3. *Help children develop reparative skills.* Feelings of guilt typically motivate a desire to fix or repair the harm that was done. But making things right is often more easily said than done. This is especially challenging for young children, who have yet to develop the complex social

and problem-solving skills necessary to formulate an effective plan for reparation. Parents can be of great help by talking the situation through, helping children identify the specific negative consequences of their actions and assisting them to devise appropriate strategies to take reparative action. After all, the ultimate goal of "moral" thought and emotion is to make things right and/or make positive changes for the future. In this way, parents can teach their children to resolve feelings of guilt effectively by proactively making themselves better people and the world a better place.

4. *Avoid public humiliation.* On the one hand, discipline is most effective when given immediately—"in the moment." On the other hand, there is the very real possibility of shaming the child, especially in settings where social approval is important (e.g., with peers). As we have emphasized, shamed children are not particularly likely to own up to their faults and "make things right." Parents can avoid unnecessarily shaming their child by adopting a respectful manner and being sensitive to the immediate social setting.

5. *Avoid teasing, derisive humor.* Sarcastic humor is another potent but often unrecognized source of shame. There's a fine line between laughing *at* a child and laughing *with* him or her. While shared humor and lighthearted teasing may add levity to a situation, humor can take a turn for the worse. Children are sensitive. It's not unusual for jokes meant in fun to be interpreted as a put-down, leading to a sense of being mocked, ridiculed, and shamed.

6. *Place discipline in a nurturing context.* It's easy for parents to get caught up in the day-to-day business of discipline. Children typically need lots of it. And sometimes parents may feel that they do little else than remind, scold, and reprimand. But, to thrive, children also need much love and affection. Again, it's important to remember that discipline is most effective when it is delivered in the context of a mutually respectful and loving relationship. *Positive* feedback is at least as important as negative feedback. In fact, research has shown that *positive* reinforcement is one of the most powerful sources of learning.

The Dynamics of Shame in the Parent–Child Relationship

Regardless of their success in other areas of life, parenting is a context in which people often question their abilities and judge themselves harshly. So it's worth mentioning that children are not the only ones in the family who are vulnerable to shame. A parent's shame can arise from many sources. Mothers and fathers may feel ashamed of being what they regard as "bad parents"—for losing their temper, for having selfish thoughts, for not providing their children with "enough." In addition to their own expectations, parents are faced with the expectations and standards of others. They may feel judged unfavorably by their spouse, by their own parents, by teachers, or by the world at large—shamed for not being the kind of parents they should be.

Parents may be especially vulnerable to feeling shame when their children misbehave, fail, or transgress. Many people regard their children's behavior as a direct reflection on themselves as parents. What parent has not felt at least an occasional painful blast of shame or embarrassment when their child has thrown a temper tantrum in the grocery line, picked their nose on stage for the entire first act of the school play, or behaved obnoxiously with someone else's apparently well-mannered (and well-parented) child? Parents may find it helpful to remember that there is no such thing as the "perfect parent"—nor the "shame-free" parent. These feelings come with the territory of parenting.

What's more important is how parents handle their feelings of shame. Throughout this book, we have emphasized many of the negative consequences of shame—withdrawal, denial, difficulties with empathy, externalization of blame, and anger. Each of these reactions can have a direct impact on parents' interactions with their children. A critical step toward circumventing these shame-related problems is simply to recognize and acknowledge those feelings of shame. Shame has its most corrosive effect when hidden and denied.

In parenting, it is especially important to remember the link between shame and anger. When people feel shamed as parents, they often feel angry with their children—whether the children deserve it or not. Moreover, shame typically leads to a hostile, irrational, destructive type of anger. Parents can benefit from this insight by taking disproportionate anger as a cue to step back and take a second look. Is there some underlying element of shame or embarrassment fueling this anger? The simple recognition of a hidden shame can put the situation in perspective. In any event, a "parental time-out" can be enormously helpful in sorting out an appropriate and constructive response.

Finally, the link between shame and anger pertains to children as well as parents. When faced with a furious, enraged child, parents may find it helpful to consider whether underlying feelings of shame are fueling the child's anger. Like adults, children are inclined to react to the discomfort of shame with externalization of blame and anger. But, developmentally, children have fewer resources to control their experience and expression of shame-based feelings of rage. In such instances, attempts to address a child's humiliated fury rationally ("Why are you so angry? What you're saying doesn't really make sense . . . ") may only cause the situation to escalate. Instead, parents can help by zeroing in on the child's initial feeling of shame and empathizing with the underlying fear and discomfort. As we have already mentioned, feelings of shame are often diffused simply by bringing them out in the open. By helping the child recognize shame as the root of his or her anger, parents can guide the child toward a more productive and rational discussion of how best to handle the anger-eliciting situation.

IMPLICATIONS FOR TEACHERS: SHAME IN THE CLASSROOM

Children spend a large portion of their childhood in school, learning new skills in both the academic and the social realms. They are there to learn things that they don't know. As a consequence, this context of new challenges and experiences has great potential for causing shame. Faced with unfamiliar territory, setbacks and failure are inevitable. Moreover, the stakes are typically quite high. At school, children grapple daily with challenges in two key contexts central to an emerging sense of self-worth. In our society, what is more important to a school-age child than doing well in school and having friends?

Learning and failure go hand in hand, and an important part of a child's education is learning how to cope effectively with failure. Failure is unpleasant for everyone, but (as highlighted by the work of Carol S. Dweck and E. L. Leggett, 1988) there are good ways and bad ways to experience failure. Some children tackle new tasks, fail, and search for new information and strategies to get it right the second time around. Their focus is on the challenge of the new task, not on themselves. Other children focus less on the task and more on the failure and its implications for their developing sense of self-worth. These children are more likely to experience shame. They are more likely to become "stuck" in shameful feelings of worthlessness and powerlessness. In fact, shame can seriously undermine children's ability to learn in a challenging environment by lessening their chance of success in future endeavors. Feeling shame, children often simply stop trying.

How can teachers provide a safe environment for children to tackle new challenges and experience inevitable failures without the destructive consequences of shame? Much of the previous discussion of guilt-inducing, shame-reducing parenting strategies apply to the classroom as well. In this regard, it is useful for teachers to keep in mind the critical distinction between guilt about specific behaviors, on the one hand, and shame about the self, on the other. Teachers can minimize students' experiences of shame by focusing on the behavior, not the person, when giving negative feedback: "John, we don't allow hitting," as opposed to "John, you're a bully"; or "Sara, you made some mistakes on the subtraction section," rather than "Sara, you're certainly no mathematician!"

Owing to their very nature, some disciplinary strategies are more shame provoking than others. Common practices that ultimately result in public humiliation and shame include writing the names of students on the chalkboard (because of misbehavior or poor performance), punishing students by making them stand up in front of the class to be chastised (often experienced as a form of ridicule), and putting students in the corner.

Teachers can further reduce shame in the classroom by discouraging children from shaming their classmates. Peers play an important role in providing feedback to children about what kinds of behaviors are socially appropriate. However, excessive amounts of teasing, criticism, and ridicule are destructive to children's developing sense of self. By monitoring and discouraging shaming interactions, teachers can help create an emotionally safe environment in which classmates can learn from one another.

An overemphasis on academic competition can create unintended consequences. While it is important to enhance students' academic motivation, it's also important to recognize that students come to the classroom with differing levels of ability and family support. Teachers may inadvertently induce painful feelings of shame by adopting practices such as making grades conspicuously public, overplaying the honor role at the expense of other students' efforts and accomplishments, and indiscriminately setting goals that amount to unrealistic expectations for some students.

We should emphasize that in encouraging teachers to minimize shame in the classroom, we are not suggesting that teachers eliminate experiences of failure. Children need to develop skills to manage failure because failure is an inevitable part of life. Typically, when we try something new, attempt to learn additional skills, or otherwise aim for excellence, we initially fail. In fact, the only way to avoid failure is to avoid anything difficult or unfamiliar. Thus, for better or worse, failure is an integral part of the learning process. Good learners persevere in the face of failure and learn from their mistakes. In fact, children who learn this skill early on are better equipped to deal with inevitable experiences of failure throughout life. As emphasized by Carol S. Dweck (Dweck & Leggett, 1988), children benefit from learning to view failure as an important source of information about how to master a task, rather than as a reflection of their ability or worth.

Finally, teachers can benefit from recognizing their own propensity for shame. Like everyone else, teachers are human and have inevitable areas of vulnerability. But, in addition, there are some special areas of vulnerability that may arise owing to their role as teachers. For example, there's a general expectation that teachers will provide an exemplary model to their students. As teachers and scholars, they are expected to be infinitely patient, wise, and knowledgeable in all areas. These expectations are so fundamental that it is almost assumed that teachers have no life outside of the classroom. (In fact, it's not uncommon for young children to presume that their teacher literally lives at school—that school is his or her home.) But, of course, just like everyone else, teachers don't know everything. They sometimes lose patience. They are occasionally unwise. In the face of inevitable human (often public) lapses, teachers may be especially prone to experience shame because of the high expectations that come with being a teacher.

Society's expectations of teachers have expanded even further in recent years. In addition to their educational mission, teachers may at times find themselves in the role of "surrogate parent." They may be called upon to teach basic social skills, provide warmth and nurturance, and serve as the child's primary disciplinary figure. All in all, many teachers face the impossible task of being teacher, parent, and moral guide—often with a lack of parental support, and sometimes in the face of parental opposition. Such parent–teacher conflict is another potent source of shame, both for the parent and the teacher. Parents often feel shamed by their children's problematic behavior and/or by their own shortcomings as parents. And it's not uncommon for these shamed parents to then shift the shame and blame to the teacher. An awareness and understanding of the dynamics of shame can help teachers work more effectively with parents as well as students. And this awareness can help teachers cope with the many stresses and demands of their important role in children's lives.

IMPLICATIONS FOR SOCIETY:
THE CRIMINAL JUSTICE SYSTEM

Parents and teachers can do much on the front end to help kids follow a moral path. But what can we as a society do for those who stray from that moral path? A consideration of shame, guilt, and empathy has important implications in the context of crime and recidivism. Theoretically, these moral emotions are presumed to play a key role in deterring immoral and antisocial behavior while also fostering corrective change following a transgression. It is surprising, then, that the research on criminology and recidivism has devoted little attention to "moral" emotions.

The High Cost of Crime

Without question, this is an area where the stakes are extremely high. Crime is one of the leading problems in the United States, and most Americans agree it is a problem we are not handling very well. Criminal activity in 1999 cost the United States some $122 billion annually—and this figure only captures the monetary cost; each one of the 15,533 murders, the 89,107 rapes, the 916,383 assaults, the 2,099,739 burglaries left indelible marks on the lives of the victims and their loved ones. As many victims can attest, the psychological costs of crime are often far higher than the steep economic costs.

The cost of crime does not end there. Americans pay a second time around in cases where offenders are apprehended, convicted, and sentenced to serve time. Currently, the United States incarcerates a larger percentage of its population than any other developed country in the world except Russia. In fact, we incarcerate our citizens at a rate 5–10 times that of most industrialized nations. In the late 1990s, some 1.7 million Americans were behind bars—a 132% increase in one decade. At this rate, 1 of every 20 Americans born in 1997 will spend some time incarcerated, including 1 of every 11 men and 1 of 4 male African Americans.

It costs more to send someone to jail than it does to send him or her to college. In 1996, the average cost of housing an inmate in the United States was $19,655 per year. Costs vary somewhat depending on the state in which the inmate is incarcerated and whether the inmate is housed in a state prison or a local jail. State inmates housed in local jails (an increasingly common practice nationally) cost that county or city upward of $29,000 per year, due to high costs in maintaining smaller facilities.

Upon release, inmates don't receive a college degree and the corresponding opportunity to contribute to our gross national product (GNP), or the tax base, for that matter. Rather, they have a two in three chance of being reincarcerated, either by committing a new offense or by having violated probation or parole. Nationally, the recidivism rate was 62% in 1997.

As the dollar cost mounts, so too does the human cost. Of the 1.7 million Americans incarcerated, 1.4 million are parents of 2.4 million children. This translates to 1 out of 50 children in the United States growing up today with a parent absent due to incarceration. And the cycle continues—compared to their peers, those 2.4 million children of prisoners are five to six times more likely to become incarcerated themselves, sometime in the future.

Factors That Predict Recidivism: Much Water under the Bridge

As just noted, having served their sentence, two-thirds of ex-inmates reoffend and return to life behind bars. One-third are successfully reintegrated into the community—at least for the first few years after release. What distinguishes these two groups, and how can we foster a higher rate of reform?

Researchers have carefully considered factors that contribute to reform versus recidivism (D. A. Andrews & Bonta, 1994; Blackburn, 1993; Gendreau, Little, & Goggin, 1996; G. T. Harris, Rice, & Quinsey, 1993; Zamble & Quinsey, 1997). It is noteworthy that the majority of proven predictors of recidivism represent "water under the bridge"—background factors rooted in past history (unstable family life, early separation from a parent, elementary school adjustment, age of first arrest, etc.) and enduring aspects of the person (intelligence, temperament, etc.). In addition, alcohol and substance abuse, deficient education, poor employment history, and prior probation or parole violations predict repeated offense. These factors may suggest avenues of broad and difficult social change that might benefit generations far into the future. But, as Zamble and Quinsey (1997) pointed out, such static or "tombstone" factors do not provide points of intervention for the 1.7 million inmates in our prisons and jails, nor for the millions of Americans who will be newly incarcerated in this year and beyond. Their history is already written.

Shame and Guilt in the Criminal Justice System

Have any critical "here and now" dynamic factors been overlooked in past efforts to understand patterns of criminal behavior and to rehabilitate offenders? Moral emotional style is one such factor that potentially could be harnessed and enhanced to reduce the likelihood of reoffense, motivating instead a constructive, rewarding, responsible path through life. How can our society construct social and legal consequences to foster better moral emotions and outcome? Several directions come to mind:

First, our research on shame and guilt has implications for intervention strategies with criminal offenders. Efforts to treat offenders may be substantially enhanced by an explicit (not very expensive) consideration of shame and guilt. A number of innovative programs exist which draw on a restorative justice model. Restorative justice is a philosophical framework that calls for active participation by the victim, the offender, and the community with the aim of repairing the community. For example, the Impact of Crime Workshop implemented in the Adult Detention Center in Fairfax County, Virginia, emphasizes principles of community, personal responsibility, and reparation. Utilizing cognitive restructuring techniques, case workers and group facilitators challenge common distorted ways of thinking about crime, victims, and the locus of responsibility. In this population, it is not unusual for inmates to make external attributions for the cause of their conviction (e.g., an overzealous cop, an associate's betrayal, lack of employment). Another common cognitive distortion among inmates centers on the experiences of a victim. Many offenders view a broad range of crimes as "victimless." They may believe that a victim (e.g., of burglary, fraud, even rape) is not really harmed unless there is concrete physical injury. They may be oblivious to the reality of psychological pain. In a rational and supportive environment, staff assist offenders in reevaluating such notions and assumptions.

As inmates grapple with issues of responsibility, the question of blame inevitably arises. And so, too, do the emotions of self-blame. Upon reexamining the causes of their legal difficulties and revisiting the circumstances surrounding the offense and its consequences, many inmates experience new feelings of shame or guilt, or both. Another important feature of the restorative justice approach is its guilt-inducing, shame-reducing philosophy and associated methods. Cognitive-behavioral interventions aimed at fostering an adaptive capacity for moral emotions include (1) educating offenders about the distinction between feelings of guilt about specific behaviors and feelings of shame about the self, (2) encouraging appropriate experiences of guilt and emphasizing associated constructive motivations to repair or make amends, (3) helping offenders recognize and modify maladaptive shame experiences, and (4) using inductive and educational strategies to foster a capacity for perspective taking and other-oriented empathy.

A second critical area where basic research on moral emotions has immediate applied implications concerns judicial sentencing practices. As the costs of incarceration mount and evidence of its failure as a deterrent grows, judges understandably have begun to search for creative alternatives to traditional sentences. One recent trend is the use of "shaming" sentences—sanctions explicitly designed to induce feelings of shame. Judges across the country are sentencing offenders to parade around in public carrying signs broadcasting their crimes, to post signs on their front lawns warning neighbors of their vices, and to display "drunk driver" bumper stickers on their cars. In our view, this is a woefully misguided approach, given the many drawbacks of shame that have been documented in the literature, in contrast to the considerable benefits of guilt.

On a more positive note, other judges have focused on sentencing alternatives based on a restorative justice model. From this perspective, crime is viewed as a violation of the victim and the community, not a violation of the state. There is an emphasis on offenders taking responsibility for their crimes and then acting to repair the harm caused to the victim and community. Thus, the ultimate aim of restorative justice is to repair the fabric of the community, rather than punishment for its own sake. Sentences in the spirit of restorative justice, such as community service, are more apt to foster feelings of guilt for the offense and its consequences, rather than feelings of shame and humiliation about the self.[1] In addition, these measures add *to* society, rather than taking *from* society (e.g., the costs of incarceration).

A consideration of shame and guilt also has implication for jail and prison policies and procedures. Aspects of the incarceration experience itself may provoke feelings of shame and humiliation. Research suggests that, particularly when punishment is perceived as unjust, such feelings of shame can lead to defiance and, paradoxically, an increase in criminal behavior (Sherman, 1993). This is especially troubling in light of Indermaur's (1994) finding that fully 90% of offenders view their sentences as unfair. A thoughtful examination of the prison environment and policies could substantially reduce the shaming, humiliating potential of life behind bars, shifting the emphasis toward values of responsibility and community.

SUMMARY AND CONCLUSIONS

In this chapter, we have discussed some of the applied implications of our research for parents and teachers who wish to foster healthy moral development in children. In particular, we offer some specific suggestions on how parents and teachers might adopt a guilt-inducing, shame-reducing strategy for responding to children's misdeeds and failures. Our findings regarding shame and guilt also have implications for the criminal justice system. Specifically, new insights into the nature and functions of these moral emotions can help enhance interventions with offenders, judicial sentencing practices, prison policy and procedures, and the prediction of violent and nonviolent recidivism.

Our book's "take-home" message—broadly applicable in many contexts—is that there are good ways and bad ways to feel bad in response to the inevitable failures and transgressions of everyday life. Shame and guilt are frequently mentioned in the same breath, but more than a decade of research underscores that these are distinct emotions, with very different implications for our personal well-being, for our relationships with others, and for society at large. Although shame and guilt are both generally regarded as "moral" emotions, they are not equally moral or adaptive. Guilt appears to lead people in a constructive, other-oriented direction. Shame, in contrast, is a moral emotion that can easily go awry. Our lives as individuals, as social beings, and as a society can be enhanced by transforming painful, problematic feelings of shame into more adaptive feelings of guilt. Recognizing the distinction between shame and guilt is an important first step in making ours a more moral society.

NOTE

1. It should be noted that Braithwaite's (1989) concept of "reintegrative shaming" shares little in common with the "shaming" sentencing practices gaining prevalence in the United States. Instead, reintegrative shaming falls squarely into the latter, restorative justice model. As detailed in Braithwaite and Mugford (1994), reintegrative shaming identifies the *crime* (behavior), not the individual, as irresponsible, wrong, or bad. In fact in this scheme, self and behavior are explicitly "uncoupled" so that the "self of the perpetrator is sustained as sacred rather than profane" (p. 146). This focus on behavior, not person, together with Braithwaite's emphasis on apology and remediation, seems much more congruent with the dynamics of *guilt*. Braithwaite and his colleagues (Braithwaite & Mugsford, 1994; Mugsford & Mugsford, 1991) have pioneered an innovative set of procedures designed to induce what sounds more like guilt (as opposed to shame) in an effort to constructively reintegrate offenders back into the community. Unfortunately, use of the term "shaming" is apt to perpetuate the confusion between shame and guilt already so prevalent in the literature. As stressed by several criminologists (Karp, 1998; Massaro, 1997; Vagg, 1998), there is good reason to expect shaming sentences, *aimed at inducing feelings of humiliation and shame about the self*, to be *disintegrative* not reintegrative—stigmatizing, isolating, excluding the offender, and ultimately increasing the likelihood of reoffense.

Appendix A

TABLES OF FINDINGS FROM
STUDIES OF SHAME AND GUILT

TABLE A.1. Adults' Phenomenological Ratings of Personal Shame and Guilt Experiences

Dimension	Shame	Guilt	t-Value
Felt bad during experience	6.41 (0.84)	5.95 (1.28)	2.37*
Writing situation was difficult	3.79 (2.13)	3.31 (1.81)	1.71*
The emotion had a sudden onset	4.94 (2.12)	4.44 (2.02)	1.44
Time moved quickly	2.59 (1.84)	3.43 (1.89)	2.63**
The emotion lasted a short time	2.46 (1.70)	2.81 (1.76)	1.23
Felt people were looking at me	5.30 (1.83)	4.22 (2.02)	3.79***
Focused on what I thought of myself (vs. others' opinions)	3.11 (2.23)	4.02 (2.30)	2.50**
Felt isolated from others	5.19 (1.70)	4.22 (1.84)	3.48***
Felt physically smaller	5.24 (1.56)	4.76 (1.47)	1.99*
Felt inferior to others	5.43 (1.36)	4.65 (1.52)	3.83***
Desire to hide	5.86 (1.37)	4.89 (1.74)	4.62***
Wanted to admit what I'd done	2.73 (1.85)	3.15 (2.05)	1.94*
Desire to make amends	4.68 (2.21)	5.11 (1.79)	1.37
Felt I had violated a moral standard	4.87 (2.21)	4.17 (2.29)	2.41[a]
Wished I had acted differently	5.90 (1.72)	5.33 (2.23)	1.70
Felt responsible for what happened	6.00 (1.65)	5.84 (1.54)	0.66
Felt in control of the situation	2.48 (1.67)	3.46 (2.18)	2.90**
Physical changes (sweating, blushing)	4.87 (1.95)	4.48 (2.20)	1.18
Viewed my actions (vs. self) as bad	4.66 (2.13)	4.50 (2.13)	0.49
Knew the reasoning behind my actions	4.40 (2.30)	4.68 (2.22)	0.78
My feelings (vs. thoughts) were important	4.78 (1.86)	4.68 (1.73)	0.40
Memory of event was more auditory (vs. visual)	2.73 (1.90)	2.87 (1.79)	0.46

Note. n = 61–63. Items were rated on a 1–7 scale. Adapted from Tangney (1993b). Copyright 1993 by John Wiley & Sons, Inc. Adapted by permission.

[a]For this item, shame and guilt differed in a direction opposite from the a priori hypothesis, the magnitude of which would have been beyond chance (two-tailed).

*p < .05, **p < .01, ***p < .001, one-tailed.

TABLE A.2. Correlations of Self-Esteem with Shame and Guilt

		Bivariate correlations		Part correlations	
		Shame	Guilt	Shame residuals	Guilt residuals
Self-esteem					
Child studies					
Study 1c—Harter	$n = 108$	−.38***	−.12	−.44***	.25**
Study 2c—Harter	$n = 317$	−.24***	.04	−.29***	.17**
Study 3c—Harter	$n = 361$	−.24***	−.02	−.26***	.09
Adolescent studies					
Study 1a—Coopersmith	$n = 440$	−.48***	−.15**	−.46***	.05
Undergraduate studies					
Study 1—Janis Field	$n = 181–182$	−.46***	−.08	−.48***	.13
Study 1—Rosenberg	$n = 182–183$	−.38***	−.01	−.42***	.17*
Study 2—Rosenberg	$n = 265$	−.43***	−.09	−.44***	.12
Study 3—Rosenberg	$n = 248–254$	−.31***	.01	−.37***	.20**
Study 4—Rosenberg (females)	$n = 200$	−.41***	.02	−.46***	.22**
Study 4—Rosenberg (males)	$n = 200$	−.32***	−.06	−.32***	.07
Study 5—Rosenberg	$n = 244$	−.38***	.06	−.42***	.20**
Study 6—Rosenberg	$n = 350$	−.46***	−.09	−.47***	.13*
Study 7—Rosenberg	$n = 86$	−.39***	−.13	−.37***	.04
Stability of self-esteem					
Undergraduate studies					
Study 1—Rosenberg	$n = 182–183$	−.36***	−.08	−.36***	.07
Study 2—Rosenberg	$n = 265$	−.36***	−.10	−.35***	.07
Study 3—Rosenberg	$n = 248–254$	−.36***	−.07	−.38***	.14*
Study 4—Rosenberg (females)	$n = 200$	−.24**	.08	−.31***	.21**
Study 4—Rosenberg (males)	$n = 200$	−.29***	.06	−.34***	.20**
Study 5—Rosenberg	$n = 244$	−.26***	.08	−.31***	.18**
Study 6—Rosenberg	$n = 350$	−.36***	−.08	−.36***	.09
Study 7—Rosenberg	$n = 86$	−.24*	.07	−.30**	.19

Note. *p < .05, **p < .01, ***p < .001, one-tailed.

TABLE A.3. Correlations of Empathy with Shame and Guilt

		Bivariate correlations		Part correlations	
		Shame	Guilt	Shame residuals	Guilt residuals
Interpersonal Reactivity Index					
Perspective taking					
Study 1—Adolescents	$n = 443$	.13**	.46***	-.06	.45***
Study 2—College Students	$n = 197$	-.01	.34***	-.13	.37***
Study 3—College Students	$n = 251$	.04	.34***	-.15*	.37***
Study 4—College Students	$n = 265$	.07	.26***	-.06	.26***
Study 5—College Students	$n = 214$ (males)	.04	.39***	-.13	.41***
Study 5—College Students	$n = 215$ (females)	-.04	.23**	-.16*	.28***
Study 6—College Students	$n = 244$	-.03	.26***	-.12	.28***
Study 7—College Students	$n = 380$	.08	.33***	-.07	.33***
Study 8—Adults	$n = 192$	-.05	.29***	-.19*	.34***
Empathic concern					
Study 1—Adolescents	$n = 442$	.24***	.54***	.02	.48***
Study 2—College Students	$n = 197$	.17*	.49***	.01	.46***
Study 3—College Students	$n = 251$	.15*	.45***	-.09	.43***
Study 4—College Students	$n = 265$	.20**	.40***	.02	.35***
Study 5—College Students	$n = 214$ (males)	.17*	.42***	-.01	.39***
Study 5—College Students	$n = 215$ (females)	.06	.30***	-.09	.31***
Study 6—College Students	$n = 243$	.17**	.45***	.02	.42***
Study 7—College Students	$n = 380$	.22***	.44***	.03	.38***
Study 8—Adults	$n = 193$	.11	.33***	-.04	.32***
Personal distress					
Study 1—Adolescents	$n = 443$	.40***	.32***	.30***	.17***
Study 2—College Students	$n = 197$	.42***	.04	.44***	-.11
Study 3—College Students	$n = 251$	.34***	.13*	.31***	-.05
Study 4—College Students	$n = 265$	.41***	.17**	.38***	-.02

(continued)

TABLE A.3. (continued)

		Bivariate correlations		Part correlations	
		Shame	Guilt	Shame residuals	Guilt residuals
Study 5—College Students	n = 214 (males)	.46***	.06	.48***	−.14*
Study 5—College Students	n = 215 (females)	.31***	.15*	.26***	.02
Study 6—College Students	n = 244	.37***	.01	.39***	−.12
Study 7—College Students	n = 380	.47***	.22***	.41***	.02
Study 8—Adults	n = 193	.42***	.14	.40***	−.05
Fantasy					
Study 1—Adolescents	n = 443	.24***	.28***	.14**	.20***
Study 2—College Students	n = 197	.12	.22**	.06	.18*
Study 3—College Students	n = 251	.15*	.22***	.05	.16**
Study 4—College Students	n = 265	.17**	.26***	.06	.20**
Study 5—College Students	n = 214 (males)	.23**	.23**	.15*	.15*
Study 5—College Students	n = 215 (females)	.08	.16*	.01	.14*
Study 6—College Students	n = 244	.20**	.18**	.14*	.12
Study 7—College Students	n = 380	.22***	.22***	.13**	.14**
Study 8—Adults	n = 193	.33***	.18*	.28***	.05
Feshbach—Adult					
General empathy					
Study 3—College Students	n = 182–183	.32***	.42***	.15*	.32***
Study 4—College Students	n = 252	.26***	.45***	.04	.37***
Study 5—College Students	n = 215 (males)	.26***	.34***	.14*	.26***
Study 5—College Students	n = 216 (females)	.20**	.32***	.06	.26***
Study 6—College Students	n = 244	.13*	.46***	−.02	.44***
Cognitive empathy					
Study 3—College Students	n = 182–183	−.08	.24**	−.20**	.31***
Study 4—College Students	n = 252	−.01	.26***	−.16*	.30***
Study 5—College Students	n = 215 (males)	−.09	.33***	−.24***	.40***
Study 5—College Students	n = 216 (females)	−.03	.14*	−.11	.17*
Study 6—College Students	n = 244	−.04	.25***	−.14*	.28***

Emotional reactivity

Study 3—College Students	n = 182–183	.11	.22**	.02	.19*
Study 4—College Students	n = 252	–.01	.19**	–.13*	.23***
Study 5—College Students	n = 215 (males)	.04	.21**	–.05	.21**
Study 5—College Students	n = 216 (females)	–.09	.18**	–.19**	.25***
Study 6—College Students	n = 244	–.10	.18**	–.17**	.22***

Affective cue recognition

Study 3—College Students	n = 182–183	–.09	.13	–.16*	.20**
Study 4—College Students	n = 252	–.09	.04	–.13*	.10
Study 5—College Students	n = 215 (males)	–.26***	.13	–.35***	.26***
Study 5—College Students	n = 216 (females)	–.12	.02	–.14*	.09
Study 6—College Students	n = 244	–.13*	.18**	–.20**	.24***

Total empathy

Study 3—College Students	n = 182–183	.12	.36***	–.04	.36***
Study 4—College Students	n = 252	.07	.33***	–.11	.34***
Study 5—College Students	n = 215 (males)	.01	.36***	–.15*	.39***
Study 5—College Students	n = 216 (females)	.01	.24***	–.11	.26***
Study 6—College Students	n = 244	–.03	.38***	–.17**	.41***

Feshbach—Child/adolescent

Affective empathy

Study 1—Children	n = 348	.27***	.36***	.13*	.28***
Study 2—Adolescents	n = 309	.38***	.44***	.18**	.30***

Cognitive empathy

Study 1—Children	n = 344	.07	.06	.05	.04
Study 2—Adolescents	n = 310	.22***	.22***	.13*	.13*

Total empathy

Study 1—Children	n = 348	.21***	.27***	.11*	.20***
Study 2—Adolescents	n = 311	.38***	.42***	.20***	.27***

Note. *p < .05, **p < .01, ***p < .001, one-tailed.

TABLE A.4. Relationship of Shame-Proneness and Guilt-Proneness to Indices of Psychopathology

	Bivariate correlations		Part correlations	
	Shame	Guilt	Shame residuals	Guilt residuals
Beck Depression Inventory				
Study 1	.28***	.02	.32***	−.15*
Study 2	.41***	.04	.45***	−.16*
Symptom Checklist-90				
Somatization				
Study 1	.28***	.06	.29***	−.10
Study 2	.33***	.06	.35***	−.10
Study 3	.20**	.06	.19**	−.03
Obsessive–Compulsive				
Study 1	.31***	.01	.36***	−.17**
Study 2	.40***	.07	.42***	−.12
Study 3	.34***	.13*	.32***	−.03
Psychoticism				
Study 1	.30***	.01	.34***	−.16**
Study 2	.38***	.09	.39***	−.08
Study 3	.29***	.11	.27***	−.03
Paranoid Ideation				
Study 1	.28***	.01	.32***	−.16**
Study 2	.35***	.08	.36***	−.08
Study 3	.26***	−.01	.30***	−.14*
Hostility–Anger				
Study 1	.10	−.17**	.22***	−.26***
Study 2	.21**	−.06	.27**	−.18*
Study 3	.05	−.11	.12	−.15*
Interpersonal Sensitivity				
Study 1	.39***	.08	.41***	−.14*
Study 2	.42***	.12	.42***	−.08
Study 3	.36***	.12	.34***	−.05
Anxiety				
Study 1	.28***	.09	.27***	−.06
Study 2	.37***	.12	.36***	−.05
Study 3	.25***	.06	.25***	−.06
Phobic Anxiety				
Study 1	.28***	.06	.29***	−.10
Study 2	.31***	.02	.34***	−.14
Study 3	.18**	−.02	.21***	−.11
Depression				
Study 1	.36***	.09	.37***	−.12
Study 2	.43***	.11	.44***	−.09
Study 3	.36***	.07	.37***	−.11

Note. Study 1, n = 253–254; Study 2, n = 158; Study 3, n = 252. All subjects were college undergraduates at a large public university.

*p < .05, **p < .01, ***p < .001.

TABLE A.5. Stabilities of Children's Shame-Proneness and Guilt-Proneness over an 8-Year Period

Moral emotion	Age 10 with age 12	Age 12 with age 18	Age 10 with age 18
Shame	.32***	.38***	.23***
Guilt	.31***	.41***	.31***
Shame residual	.27***	.37***	.19***
Guilt residual	.26***	.40***	.27***
(n)	(246)	(200)	(261)

Note. ***p < .001, one-tailed.

TABLE A.6. Stabilities of Parents' and Grandparents' Shame-Proneness and Guilt-Proneness over a 2-Year Period

Sample	Shame	Guilt	Shame residuals	Guilt residuals	(n)
Mothers	.71***	.53***	.71***	.52***	(152)
Fathers	.65***	.49***	.64***	.48***	(115)
Maternal grandmothers	.73***	.56***	.64***	.46***	(101)
Paternal grandmothers	.73***	.39***	.66***	.34***	(80)
Maternal grandfathers	.63***	.32**	.53***	.27*	(64)
Paternal grandfathers	.59***	.43**	.59***	.43**	(45)

Note. *p < .05, **p < .01, ***p < .001, one-tailed.

Appendix B

MEASURES OF SHAME AND GUILT

TEST OF SELF-CONSCIOUS AFFECT–3 (TOSCA-3)

Below are situations that people are likely to encounter in day-to-day life, followed by several common reactions to those situations.

As you read each scenario, try to imagine yourself in that situation. Then indicate how likely you would be to react in each of the ways described. We ask you to rate *all* responses because people may feel or react more than one way to the same situation, or they may react different ways at different times.

For example:

You wake up early one Saturday morning. It is cold and rainy outside.

a) You would telephone a friend to catch up on news.

    ①- 2 - - 3 - - 4 - - 5
    not likely   very likely

b) You would take the extra time to read the paper.

    1 - - 2 - - 3 - - 4 - ⑤
    not likely   very likely

c) You would feel disappointed that it's raining.

    1 - - 2 - ③ - 4 - - 5
    not likely   very likely

d) You would wonder why you woke up so early.

    1 - - 2 - - 3 - ④ - 5
    not likely   very likely

In the above example, I've rated *all* of the answers by circling a number. I circled a "1" for answer (a) because I wouldn't want to wake up a friend very early on a Saturday morning—so it's not at all likely that I would do that. I circled a "5" for answer (b) because I almost always read the paper if I have time in the morning (very likely). I circled a "3" for answer (c) because for me it's about half and half. Sometimes I would be disappointed about the rain and sometimes I wouldn't—it would depend on what I had planned. And I circled a "4" for answer (d) because I would probably wonder why I had awakened so early.

Please do not skip any items—rate all responses.

1. *You make plans to meet a friend for lunch. At 5 o'clock, you realize you stood your friend up.*

    a) You would think: "I'm inconsiderate."

        1 - - 2 - - 3 - - 4 - - 5
        not likely   very likely

    b) You would think: "Well, my friend will understand."

        1 - - 2 - - 3 - - 4 - - 5
        not likely   very likely

c) You'd think you should make it up to your
friend as soon as possible.

$1 - - 2 - - 3 - - 4 - - 5$
not likely   very likely

d) You would think: "My boss distracted me
just before lunch."

$1 - - 2 - - 3 - - 4 - - 5$
not likely   very likely

2. *You break something at work and then hide it.*

a) You would think: "This is making me
anxious. I need to either fix it or get
someone else to."

$1 - - 2 - - 3 - - 4 - - 5$
not likely   very likely

b) You would think about quitting.

$1 - - 2 - - 3 - - 4 - - 5$
not likely   very likely

c) You would think: "A lot of things aren't
made very well these days."

$1 - - 2 - - 3 - - 4 - - 5$
not likely   very likely

d) You would think: "It was only an accident."

$1 - - 2 - - 3 - - 4 - - 5$
not likely   very likely

3. *You are out with friends one evening, and you're feeling especially witty and*
attractive. Your best friend's spouse seems to particularly enjoy your com-
pany.

a) You would think: "I should have been
aware of what my best friend was feeling."

$1 - - 2 - - 3 - - 4 - - 5$
not likely   very likely

b) You would feel happy with your
appearance and personality.

$1 - - 2 - - 3 - - 4 - - 5$
not likely   very likely

c) You would feel pleased to have made
such a good impression.

$1 - - 2 - - 3 - - 4 - - 5$
not likely   very likely

d) You would think your best friend should
pay attention to his/her spouse.

$1 - - 2 - - 3 - - 4 - - 5$
not likely   very likely

e) You would probably avoid eye contact
for a long time.

$1 - - 2 - - 3 - - 4 - - 5$
not likely   very likely

4. *At work, you wait until the last minute to plan a project, and it turns out*
badly.

a) You would feel incompetent.

$1 - - 2 - - 3 - - 4 - - 5$
not likely   very likely

b) You would think: "There are never enough
hours in the day."

$1 - - 2 - - 3 - - 4 - - 5$
not likely   very likely

c) You would feel: "I deserve to be reprimanded for mismanaging the project."

1 - - 2 - - 3 - - 4 - - 5
not likely   very likely

d) You would think: "What's done is done."

1 - - 2 - - 3 - - 4 - - 5
not likely   very likely

5. *You make a mistake at work and find out a coworker is blamed for the error.*

a) You would think the company did not like the coworker.

1 - - 2 - - 3 - - 4 - - 5
not likely   very likely

b) You would think: "Life is not fair."

1 - - 2 - - 3 - - 4 - - 5
not likely   very likely

c) You would keep quiet and avoid the coworker.

1 - - 2 - - 3 - - 4 - - 5
not likely   very likely

d) You would feel unhappy and eager to correct the situation.

1 - - 2 - - 3 - - 4 - - 5
not likely   very likely

6. *For several days you put off making a difficult phone call. At the last minute you make the call and are able to manipulate the conversation so that all goes well.*

a) You would think: "I guess I'm more persuasive than I thought."

1 - - 2 - - 3 - - 4 - - 5
not likely   very likely

b) You would regret that you put it off.

1 - - 2 - - 3 - - 4 - - 5
not likely   very likely

c) You would feel like a coward.

1 - - 2 - - 3 - - 4 - - 5
not likely   very likely

d) You would think: "I did a good job."

1 - - 2 - - 3 - - 4 - - 5
not likely   very likely

e) You would think you shouldn't have to make calls you feel pressured into.

1 - - 2 - - 3 - - 4 - - 5
not likely   very likely

7. *While playing around, you throw a ball and it hits your friend in the face.*

a) You would feel inadequate that you can't even throw a ball.

1 - - 2 - - 3 - - 4 - - 5
not likely   very likely

b) You would think maybe your friend needs more practice at catching.

1 - - 2 - - 3 - - 4 - - 5
not likely   very likely

c) You would think: "It was just an accident." 1 - - 2 - - 3 - - 4 - - 5
                                                not likely   very likely

d) You would apologize and make sure your   1 - - 2 - - 3 - - 4 - - 5
   friend feels better.   not likely   very likely

8. *You have recently moved away from your family, and everyone has been very helpful. A few times you needed to borrow money, but you paid it back as soon as you could.*

   a) You would feel immature.   1 - - 2 - - 3 - - 4 - - 5
                                                not likely   very likely

   b) You would think: "I sure ran into some   1 - - 2 - - 3 - - 4 - - 5
      bad luck."   not likely   very likely

   c) You would return the favor as quickly   1 - - 2 - - 3 - - 4 - - 5
      as you could.   not likely   very likely

   d) You would think: "I am a trustworthy   1 - - 2 - - 3 - - 4 - - 5
      person."   not likely   very likely

   e) You would be proud that you repaid   1 - - 2 - - 3 - - 4 - - 5
      your debts.   not likely   very likely

9. *You are driving down the road, and you hit a small animal.*

   a) You would think the animal shouldn't   1 - - 2 - - 3 - - 4 - - 5
      have been on the road.   not likely   very likely

   b) You would think: "I'm terrible."   1 - - 2 - - 3 - - 4 - - 5
                                                not likely   very likely

   c) You would feel: "Well, it was an accident." 1 - - 2 - - 3 - - 4 - - 5
                                                not likely   very likely

   d) You'd feel bad you hadn't been more alert 1 - - 2 - - 3 - - 4 - - 5
      driving down the road.   not likely   very likely

10. *You walk out of an exam thinking you did extremely well. Then you find out you did poorly.*

    a) You would think: "Well, it's just a test." 1 - - 2 - - 3 - - 4 - - 5
                                                 not likely   very likely

    b) You would think: "The instructor doesn't 1 - - 2 - - 3 - - 4 - - 5
       like me."   not likely   very likely

c) You would think: "I should have
studied harder."

1 - - 2 - - 3 - - 4 - - 5
not likely   very likely

d) You would feel stupid.

1 - - 2 - - 3 - - 4 - - 5
not likely   very likely

11. *You and a group of coworkers worked very hard on a project. Your boss singles you out for a bonus because the project was such a success.*

a) You would feel the boss is rather
short-sighted.

1 - - 2 - - 3 - - 4 - - 5
not likely   very likely

b) You would feel alone and apart from
your colleagues.

1 - - 2 - - 3 - - 4 - - 5
not likely   very likely

c) You would feel your hard work had
paid off.

1 - - 2 - - 3 - - 4 - - 5
not likely   very likely

d) You would feel competent and proud
of yourself.

1 - - 2 - - 3 - - 4 - - 5
not likely   very likely

e) You would feel you should not accept it.

1 - - 2 - - 3 - - 4 - - 5
not likely   very likely

12. *While out with a group of friends, you make fun of a friend who's not there.*

a) You would think: "It was all in fun;
it's harmless."

1 - - 2 - - 3 - - 4 - - 5
not likely   very likely

b) You would feel small . . . like a rat.

1 - - 2 - - 3 - - 4 - - 5
not likely   very likely

c) You would think that perhaps that friend
should have been there to defend
him/herself.

1 - - 2 - - 3 - - 4 - - 5
not likely   ¦   very likely

d) You would apologize and talk about that
person's good points.

1 - - 2 - - 3 - - 4 - - 5
not likely   very likely

13. *You make a big mistake on an important project at work. People were depending on you, and your boss criticizes you.*

a) You would think your boss should have
been more clear about what was
expected of you.

1 - - 2 - - 3 - - 4 - - 5
not likely   very likely

b) You would feel like you wanted to hide.

1 - - 2 - - 3 - - 4 - - 5
not likely   very likely

c) You would think: "I should have recognized   1 - - 2 - - 3 - - 4 - - 5
the problem and done a better job."   not likely   very likely

d) You would think: "Well, nobody's perfect."   1 - - 2 - - 3 - - 4 - - 5
                                      not likely   very likely

14. *You volunteer to help with the local Special Olympics for handicapped children. It turns out to be frustrating and time-consuming work. You think
seriously about quitting, but then you see how happy the kids are.*

a) You would feel selfish, and you'd think you   1 - - 2 - - 3 - - 4 - - 5
are basically lazy.   not likely   very likely

b) You would feel you were forced into doing   1 - - 2 - - 3 - - 4 - - 5
something you did not want to do.   not likely   very likely

c) You would think: "I should be more   1 - - 2 - - 3 - - 4 - - 5
concerned about people who are less   not likely   very likely
fortunate."

d) You would feel great that you had helped   1 - - 2 - - 3 - - 4 - - 5
others.   not likely   very likely

e) You would feel very satisfied with yourself.   1 - - 2 - - 3 - - 4 - - 5
                                      not likely   very likely

15. *You are taking care of your friend's dog while your friend is on vacation,
and the dog runs away.*

a) You would think, "I am irresponsible   1 - - 2 - - 3 - - 4 - - 5
and incompetent."   not likely   very likely

b) You would think your friend must not take   1 - - 2 - - 3 - - 4 - - 5
very good care of the dog or it wouldn't   not likely   very likely
have run away.

c) You would vow to be more careful next time.   1 - - 2 - - 3 - - 4 - - 5
                                      not likely   very likely

d) You would think your friend could just get   1 - - 2 - - 3 - - 4 - - 5
a new dog.   not likely   very likely

16. *You attend your coworker's housewarming party and you spill red wine on a
new cream-colored carpet, but you think no one notices.*

a) You think your coworker should have   1 - - 2 - - 3 - - 4 - - 5
expected some accidents at such a   not likely   very likely
big party.

b) You would stay late to help clean up the stain after the party.

1 - - 2 - - 3 - - 4 - - 5
not likely   very likely

c) You would wish you were anywhere but at the party.

1 - - 2 - - 3 - - 4 - - 5
not likely   very likely

d) You would wonder why your coworker chose to serve red wine with the new light carpet.

1 - - 2 - - 3 - - 4 - - 5
not likely   very likely

We are now recommending the use of the TOSCA-3 in place of the TOSCA and TOSCA-2. The TOCSA-3 is composed of 11 negative and 5 positive scenarios yielding indices of Shame-Proneness, Guilt-Proneness, Externalization, Detachment/Unconcern, Alpha Pride, and Beta Pride.

The majority of TOSCA-3 items are identical to the original TOSCA (Tangney, Wagner, & Gramzow, 1989). TOSCA scenarios were drawn from written accounts of personal shame, guilt, and pride experiences provided by a sample of several hundred college students and noncollege adults. The responses were drawn from a much larger pool of affective, cognitive, and behavioral responses provided by a second sample of adults.

In a subsequent revision, the TOSCA-2 (Tangney, Ferguson, Wagner, Crowley, & Gramzow, 1996), an experimental "Maladaptive Guilt" scale was introduced. In addition, we added two new scenarios and deleted the "Dieting" scenario, owing to concerns about gender bias. This most recent version of our measure, the TOSCA-3 (Tangney, Dearing, Wagner, & Gramzow, 2000), eliminates the Maladaptive Guilt items because analyses have raised serious questions about the discriminant validity of this scale. (The Shame and Maladaptive Guilt scales correlate about .79.)

As a new feature, the TOSCA-3 provides the option of a short version, which drops positive scenarios (and therefore eliminates the Pride scales). In a recent study, short versions of the TOSCA-3 Shame and Guilt scales correlated .94 and .93, respectively with their corresponding full length versions, thus supporting the utility of the abbreviated form.

Scoring for the TOSCA-3*:

1. (Negative Scenario)
   a) Shame
   b) Detached
   c) Guilt
   d) Externalization
2. (Negative Scenario)
   a) Guilt

9. (Negative Scenario)
   a) Externalization
   b) Shame
   c) Detached
   d) Guilt
10. (Negative Scenario)
   a) Detached

b) Shame

c) Externalization

d) Detached

3. (Positive Scenario)

a) Guilt

b) Alpha Pride

c) Beta Pride

d) Externalization

e) Shame

4. (Negative Scenario)

a) Shame

b) Externalization

c) Guilt

d) Detached

5. (Negative Scenario)

a) Externalization

b) Detached

c) Shame

d) Guilt

6. (Positive Scenario)

a) Alpha Pride

b) Guilt

c) Shame

d) Beta Pride

e) Externalization

7. (Negative Scenario)

a) Shame

b) Externalization

c) Detached

d) Guilt

8. (Positive Scenario)

a) Shame

b) Externalization

c) Guilt

d) Alpha Pride

e) Beta Pride

b) Externalization

c) Guilt

d) Shame

11. (Positive Scenario)

a) Externalization

b) Shame

c) Beta Pride

d) Alpha Pride

e) Guilt

12. (Negative Scenario)

a) Detached

b) Shame

c) Externalization

d) Guilt

13. (Negative Scenario)

a) Externalization

b) Shame

c) Guilt

d) Detached

14. (Positive Scenario)

a) Shame

b) Externalization

c) Guilt

d) Beta Pride

e) Alpha Pride

15. (Negative Scenario)

a) Shame

b) Externalization

c) Guilt

d) Detached

16. (Negative Scenario)

a) Detached

b) Guilt

c) Shame

d) Externalization

A short version of the TOSCA-3 may be created by dropping the positive scenarios.

---

*Scale scores are the sum of responses to relevant items (e.g., the score for the Shame scale equals the respondent's answer to 1a, plus the answer to 2b, etc.).

TEST OF SELF-CONSCIOUS AFFECT
FOR ADOLESCENTS (TOSCA-A)

On the following pages, you will find descriptions of a variety of situations. After each situation, you will see several statements about different ways that people might think or feel.

As I read each situation, really imagine that you are in that situation now. Imagine how you might think or feel. After I read each statement to you, please indicate which circle describes how likely it is that the statement would be true for you. The largest circle (5) means that you are very likely to think or feel that way, and the smallest circle (1) means that you are not at all likely to think or feel that way.

For example:

You wake up early one morning on a school day.

	not at all likely	unlikely	maybe (half & half)	likely	very likely
a) I would eat breakfast right away.	①	②	⊗	④	⑤
b) I would try to do some extra chores before starting my day.	①	⊗	③	④	⑤
c) I would feel like staying in bed.	①	②	③	④	⊗
d) I would wonder why I woke up so early.	⊗	②	③	④	⑤

In the above example, I've rated *all* of the answers by putting an X in the circle. I marked "maybe" for answer (a) because there have been a few times that I have woken up early and been hungry and eaten right away. For answer (b) I marked "unlikely" because I have only woken up early and decided to do extra chores once, so it is pretty unlikely that I would do that. For answer (c) I marked "very likely" because most of the time when I wake up, I like to stay in bed for a while, so it is very likely that I would do that. For answer (d) I marked "not at all likely" because I would never wonder why I woke up so early.

There are no right or wrong answers to these questions. We're simply interested in your own thoughts and ideas about these situations.

1. *You trip in the cafeteria and spill your friend's drink.*

	not at all likely	unlikely	maybe (half & half)	likely	very likely
a) I would be thinking that everyone is watching me and laughing.	①	②	③	④	⑤
b) I would feel very sorry. I should have watched where I was going.	①	②	③	④	⑤
c) I wouldn't feel bad because it didn't cost very much.	①	②	③	④	⑤
d) I would think: "I couldn't help it. The floor was slippery."	①	②	③	④	⑤

2. *For several days you put off talking to a teacher about a missed assignment. At the last minute you talk to the teacher about it, and all goes well.*

	not at all likely	unlikely	maybe (half & half)	likely	very likely
a) I would think: "I guess I'm more convincing than I thought."	①	②	③	④	⑤
b) I would regret that I put it off.	①	②	③	④	⑤
c) I would feel like a coward.	①	②	③	④	⑤
d) I would think: "I handled that well."	①	②	③	④	⑤
e) I would think: "The teacher should have asked me about it first. It's her job."	①	②	③	④	⑤

3. *While playing around, you throw a ball and it hits your friend in the face.*

	not at all likely	unlikely	maybe (half & half)	likely	very likely
a) I would feel stupid that I can't even throw a ball.	①	②	③	④	⑤
b) I would think: "Maybe my friend needs more practice catching."	①	②	③	④	⑤

c) I would think: "It was just   ① --- ② --- ③ --- ④ --- ⑤
an accident."

d) I would apologize and make   ① --- ② --- ③ --- ④ --- ⑤
sure my friend feels better.

4. *You and a group of classmates worked very hard on a project. Your teacher singles you out for a better grade than anyone else.*

	not at all likely	unlikely	maybe (half & half)	likely	very likely
a) I would think: "The teacher is playing favorites."	①	②	③	④	⑤
b) I would feel alone and apart from my classmates.	①	②	③	④	⑤
c) I would feel that my hard work had paid off.	①	②	③	④	⑤
d) I would feel competent and proud of myself.	①	②	③	④	⑤
e) I would tell the teacher that everyone should get the same grade.	①	②	③	④	⑤

5. *You break something at a friend's house and then hide it.*

	not at all likely	unlikely	maybe (half & half)	likely	very likely
a) I would think: "This is making me anxious. I need to either fix it or replace it."	①	②	③	④	⑤
b) I would avoid seeing that friend for a while.	①	②	③	④	⑤
c) I would think: "A lot of things aren't made very well."	①	②	③	④	⑤
d) I would think: "It was only an accident."	①	②	③	④	⑤

6. *At school, you wait until the last minute to plan a project, and it turns out badly.*

	not at all likely	unlikely	maybe (half & half)	likely	very likely

a) I would feel useless and incompetent.

① - - - ② - - - ③ - - - ④ - - - ⑤

b) I would think: "There are never enough hours in the day."

① - - - ② - - - ③ - - - ④ - - - ⑤

c) I would feel that I deserve a bad grade.

① - - - ② - - - ③ - - - ④ - - - ⑤

d) I would think: "What's done is done."

① - - - ② - - - ③ - - - ④ - - - ⑤

7. *You wake up one morning and remember it's your mother's birthday. You forgot to get her something.*

	not at all likely	unlikely	maybe (half & half)	likely	very likely

a) I would think: "It's not the gift that matters. All that really matters is that I care."

① - - - ② - - - ③ - - - ④ - - - ⑤

b) I would think: "After everything she's done for me, how could I forget her birthday?"

① - - - ② - - - ③ - - - ④ - - - ⑤

c) I would feel irresponsible and thoughtless.

① - - - ② - - - ③ - - - ④ - - - ⑤

d) I would think: "Someone should have reminded me."

① - - - ② - - - ③ - - - ④ - - - ⑤

8. *You walk out of a test thinking you did extremely well. Then you find out you did poorly.*

	not at all likely	unlikely	maybe (half & half)	likely	very likely

a) I would feel that I should have done better. I should have studied more.

① - - - ② - - - ③ - - - ④ - - - ⑤

b) I would feel stupid.   ① - - - ② - - - ③ - - - ④ - - - ⑤

c) I would think: "It's only   ① - - - ② - - - ③ - - - ④ - - - ⑤
a test."

d) I would think: "The teacher   ① - - - ② - - - ③ - - - ④ - - - ⑤
must have graded it wrong."

9. *You make a mistake at school and find out a classmate is blamed for the error.*

	not at all likely	unlikely	maybe (half & half)	likely	very likely

a) I would think: "The teacher   ① - - - ② - - - ③ - - - ④ - - - ⑤
does not like the classmate."

b) I would think: "Life is   ① - - - ② - - - ③ - - - ④ - - - ⑤
not fair."

c) I would keep quiet and avoid   ① - - - ② - - - ③ - - - ④ - - - ⑤
the classmate.

d) I would feel unhappy and   ① - - - ② - - - ③ - - - ④ - - - ⑤
eager to correct the situation.

10. *You were talking in class, and your friend got blamed. You go to the teacher
and tell him the truth.*

	not at all likely	unlikely	maybe (half & half)	likely	very likely

a) I would think: "The teacher   ① - - - ② - - - ③ - - - ④ - - - ⑤
should have gotten the facts
straight before he blamed my
friend."

b) I would feel like I always   ① - - - ② - - - ③ - - - ④ - - - ⑤
get people in trouble.

c) I would feel good about   ① - - - ② - - - ③ - - - ④ - - - ⑤
setting the record straight.

d) I would be proud of myself   ① - - - ② - - - ③ - - - ④ - - - ⑤
for being an honest person.

e) I would think: "I'm the one   ① - - - ② - - - ③ - - - ④ - - - ⑤
who should get in trouble. I
shouldn't have been talking in
the first place."

11. *You and your friend are talking in class, and you get in trouble.*

	not at all likely	unlikely	maybe (half & half)	very likely	likely

a) I would think: "I should know better. I deserve to get in trouble." ① - - - ② - - - ③ - - - ④ - - - ⑤

b) I would think: "We were only whispering." ① - - - ② - - - ③ - - - ④ - - - ⑤

c) I would think: "The teacher is unfair." ① - - - ② - - - ③ - - - ④ - - - ⑤

d) I would feel like everyone in the class was looking at me and they were about to laugh. ① - - - ② - - - ③ - - - ④ - - - ⑤

12. *You make plans to meet a friend. Later you realize you stood your friend up.*

	not at all likely	unlikely	maybe (half & half)	very likely	likely

a) I would think: "I'm inconsiderate." ① - - - ② - - - ③ - - - ④ - - - ⑤

b) I would think: "Well, my friend will understand." ① - - - ② - - - ③ - - - ④ - - - ⑤

c) I would try to make it up to my friend as soon as possible. ① - - - ② - - - ③ - - - ④ - - - ⑤

d) I would think: "Someone distracted me just before I was supposed to meet my friend." ① - - - ② - - - ③ - - - ④ - - - ⑤

13. *You volunteer to help raise money for a good cause. Later you want to quit, but you know your help is important.*

	not at all likely	unlikely	maybe (half & half)	very likely	likely

a) I would feel selfish, and I'd think I am basically lazy. ① - - - ② - - - ③ - - - ④ - - - ⑤

b) I would think: "I was pressured into helping." ① - - - ② - - - ③ - - - ④ - - - ⑤

c) I would think: "I should be more concerned about doing whatever I can to help."   ① - - - ② - - - ③ - - - ④ - - - ⑤

d) I would feel great that I had helped.   ① - - - ② - - - ③ - - - ④ - - - ⑤

e) I would feel very satisfied with myself.   ① - - - ② - - - ③ - - - ④ - - - ⑤

14. *Your report card isn't as good as you wanted. You show it to your parents when you get home.*

	not at all likely	unlikely	maybe (half & half)	likely	very likely

a) I would think: "Everyone gets bad grades once in a while."   ① - - - ② - - - ③ - - - ④ - - - ⑤

b) I would think: "I really didn't deserve the grades, it wasn't my fault."   ① - - - ② - - - ③ - - - ④ - - - ⑤

c) Now that I got a bad report card, I would feel worthless.   ① - - - ② - - - ③ - - - ④ - - - ⑤

d) I would think: "I should listen to everything the teacher says and study harder."   ① - - - ② - - - ③ - - - ④ - - - ⑤

15. *You have recently moved to a new school, and everyone has been very help-ful. A few times you had to ask some big favors, but you returned the favors as soon as you could.*

	not at all likely	unlikely	maybe (half & half)	likely	very likely

a) I would feel like a failure.   ① - - - ② - - - ③ - - - ④ - - - ⑤

b) I would think: "Maybe this school doesn't do enough to help new students."   ① - - - ② - - - ③ - - - ④ - - - ⑤

c) I would be especially nice to the people who had helped me.   ① - - - ② - - - ③ - - - ④ - - - ⑤

d) I would think: "I am smart to ask for help when I need it."   ① - - - ② - - - ③ - - - ④ - - - ⑤

e) I would be proud that I returned the favors.   ① - - - ② - - - ③ - - - ④ - - - ⑤

The TOSCA-A is composed of 10 negative and 5 positive scenarios yielding indices of Shame-Proneness, Guilt-Proneness, Externalization, Detachment/Unconcern, Alpha Pride, and Beta Pride. The scenarios and associated responses were drawn in part from the TOSCA for adults and in part from the TOSCA-C for children. Some of the items were rewritten slightly to make the content more relevant for adolescents.

Scoring for the TOSCA-A*:

1. a) Shame
   b) Guilt
   c) Detached
   d) Externalization
2. a) Alpha Pride
   b) Guilt
   c) Shame
   d) Beta Pride
   e) Externalization
3. a) Shame
   b) Externalization
   c) Detached
   d) Guilt
4. a) Externalization
   b) Shame
   c) Beta Pride
   d) Alpha Pride
   e) Guilt
5. a) Guilt
   b) Shame
   c) Externalization
   d) Detached
6. a) Shame
   b) Externalization
   c) Guilt
   d) Detached
7. a) Detached
   b) Guilt
   c) Shame
   d) Externalization
8. a) Guilt
   b) Shame
   c) Detached
   d) Externalization

9. a) Externalization
   b) Detached
   c) Shame
   d) Guilt
10. a) Externalization
    b) Shame
    c) Beta Pride
    d) Alpha Pride
    e) Guilt
11. a) Guilt
    b) Detached
    c) Externalization
    d) Shame
12. a) Shame
    b) Detached
    c) Guilt
    d) Externalization
13. a) Shame
    b) Externalization
    c) Guilt
    d) Beta Pride
    e) Alpha Pride
14. a) Detached
    b) Externalization
    c) Shame
    d) Guilt
15. a) Shame
    b) Externalization
    c) Guilt
    d) Alpha Pride
    e) Beta Pride

*Scale scores are the sum of responses to relevant items (e.g., the score for the Shame scale equals the respondent's answer to 1a, plus the answer to 2c, etc.).

TEST OF SELF-CONSCIOUS AFFECT
FOR CHILDREN (TOSCA-C)

Here are some situations that might happen to you once in a while. And here are some different ways that people might think or feel.

Really imagine that you are in the situation now and imagine how you might think or feel. Then read each statement. *Put an X in the circle* to describe how likely the statement would be true for you. The largest circle means that you are very likely to think or feel that way, and the smallest circle means that you are not at all likely to respond that way.

For example:

You wake up very early one morning on a school day.

	not at all likely	unlikely	maybe (half & half)	likely	very likely
a) I would eat breakfast right away.	O	O	O	O	O
b) I would check over my homework before I left for school.	O	O	O	O	O
c) I would not feel like getting out of bed.	O	O	O	O	O

Remember that everyone has good days and bad days. Everyone sometimes does things that they wouldn't normally do. *There are no right or wrong answers to these questions.*

1. *You are on patrol duty and you turn in three kids.*

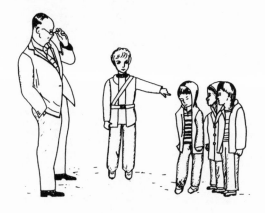

223

	not at all likely	unlikely	maybe (half & half)	likely	very likely
a) I'd worry about what would happen to them.	O	O	O	O	O
b) I'd think, "They deserved it."	O	O	O	O	O
c) I'd think, "I'm a tattletale."	O	O	O	O	O
d) I would feel good about myself.	O	O	O	O	O
e) I would feel I did a good job.	O	O	O	O	O

2. *Your aunt is giving a big party. You are carrying drinks to people, and you spill one all over the floor.*

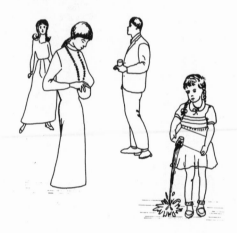

	not at all likely	unlikely	maybe (half & half)	likely	very likely
a) I should have been more careful.	O	O	O	O	O
b) My aunt wouldn't mind that much.	O	O	O	O	O
c) I would run upstairs to be away from everybody.	O	O	O	O	O
d) The tray was too heavy.	O	O	O	O	O

3. *You get a test back in school and didn't do well.*

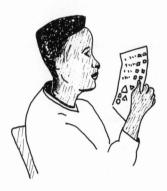

	not at all likely	unlikely	maybe (half & half)	likely	very likely
a) I'd feel that I should have done better. I should have studied more.	O	O	O	O	O
b) I'd feel stupid.	O	O	O	O	O
c) It's only one test.	O	O	O	O	O
d) The teacher must have graded it wrong.	O	O	O	O	O

4. *You stop playing all the time with one friend to play with someone who doesn't have any friends.*

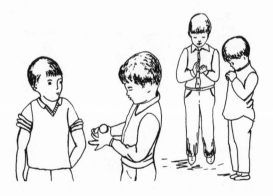

	not at all likely	unlikely	maybe (half & half)	likely	very likely
a) I'd feel bad because it's not fair to forget about one friend when you make another.	O	O	O	O	O
b) I did something good.	O	O	O	O	O
c) That new kid had lots of fun games that I wanted to play.	O	O	O	O	O
d) My other friends might think I'm weird, playing with somebody who doesn't have any friends.	O	O	O	O	O
e) I'm a really nice person to play with someone who didn't have any friends.	O	O	O	O	O

5. *You wake up one morning and remember it's your mother's birthday. You forgot to get her something.*

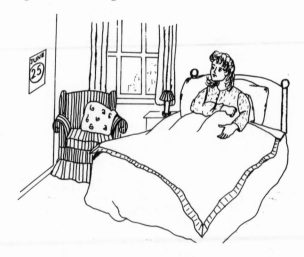

	not at all likely	unlikely	maybe (half & half)	likely	very likely
a) It's not the gift that matters. All that really matters is that I care.	O	O	O	O	O

b) After everything she's done
for me, how could I forget
her birthday?

    O   O   O   O   O

c) I would feel irresponsible
and thoughtless.

    O   O   O   O   O

d) Someone should have
reminded me.

    O   O   O   O   O

6. *You trip in the cafeteria and you spill your friend's milk.*

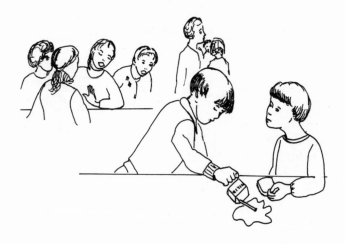

	not at all likely	unlikely	maybe (half & half)	likely	very likely
a) I'd be thinking that everyone is watching me and laughing.	O	O	O	O	O
b) I would feel sorry, very sorry. I should have watched where I was going.	O	O	O	O	O
c) I wouldn't feel bad because milk doesn't cost very much.	O	O	O	O	O
d) I couldn't help it. The floor was slippery.	O	O	O	O	O

7. *You were talking in class, and your friend got blamed. You go to the teacher and tell him the truth.*

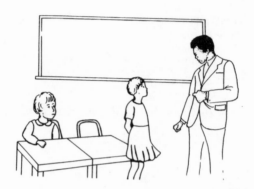

	not at all likely	unlikely	maybe (half & half)	likely	very likely
a) The teacher should have gotten the facts straight before he blamed my friend.	O	O	O	O	O
b) I would feel like I always get people in trouble.	O	O	O	O	O
c) I did a very good thing by telling the truth.	O	O	O	O	O
d) I'd be proud of myself that I'm able to tell the teacher something like that.	O	O	O	O	O
e) I'm the one who should get in trouble. I shouldn't have been talking in the first place.	O	O	O	O	O

8. *You accidentally break your aunt's vase. Your aunt scolds your little cousin instead of you.*

	not at all likely	unlikely	maybe (half & half)	likely	very likely
a) If I didn't tell the truth, something inside would bother me.	O	O	O	O	O

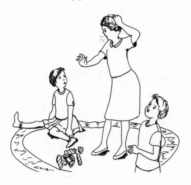

b) No one is going to like me   O   O   O   O O
   if my cousin tells on me.

c) She only scolded my cousin;   O   O   O   O O
   it's no big deal.

d) She should find out what   O   O   O   O O
   happened before she starts
   yelling.

9. *Your report card isn't as good as you wanted. You show it to your mother when you get home.*

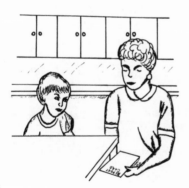

	not at all likely	unlikely	maybe (half & half)	likely	very likely
a) Everyone gets bad grades once in a while.	O	O	O	O	O
b) I really didn't deserve the grades, it wasn't my fault.	O	O	O	O	O

c) Now that I got a bad report card, I'm worthless.   O   O   O   O   O

d) I should listen to everything the teacher says and study harder.   O   O   O   O   O

10. *You and your best friend get into an argument at school.*

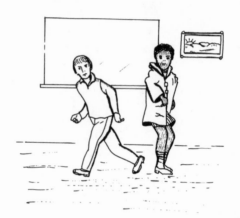

	not at all likely	unlikely	maybe (half & half)	very likely	likely
a) It was my friend's fault.	O	O	O	O	O
b) We do it all the time, and we always make up.	O	O	O	O	O
c) I would feel sorry and feel like I shouldn't have done it.	O	O	O	O	O
d) I'd probably feel real lousy about myself.	O	O	O	O	O

11. *Your teacher writes your name on the board for chewing gum in class.*

	not at all likely	unlikely	maybe (half & half)	very likely	likely
a) I'd think that my teacher was unfair to write my name on the board.	O	O	O	O	O

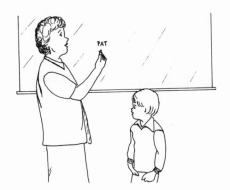

b) I'd slide down in my chair, embarrassed. ○ ○ ○ ○ ○

c) If I was chewing gum it would serve me right because it's a rule. ○ ○ ○ ○ ○

d) I wouldn't mind. People at school chew gum all the time. ○ ○ ○ ○ ○

12. *You get your report card and tell your best friend you made the honor roll. You find out your friend did not.*

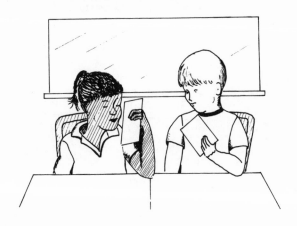

	not at all likely	unlikely	maybe (half & half)	likely	very likely
a) It's my friend's fault for not making the honor roll.	○	○	○	○	○

b) I'd feel bad because I was   ○   ○   ○   ○ ○
bragging about it and I made
my friend feel bad.

c) I'd feel good about myself for ○   ○   ○   ○ ○
being such a good student.

d) I'd be proud of my grades.   ○   ○   ○   ○ ○

e) My friend might think I'm   ○   ○   ○   ○ ○
a show-off.

13. *You and your friend are talking in class, and you get in trouble.*

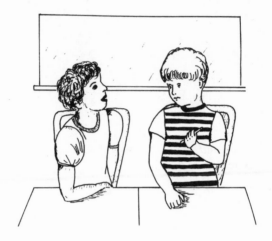

	not at all likely	unlikely	maybe (half & half)	likely	very likely
a) I'd think that I shouldn't have talked in the first place. I deserve to get in trouble.	○	○	○	○	○
b) We were only whispering.	○	○	○	○	○
c) The teacher is mean and unfair.	○	○	○	○	○
d) I'd feel like everyone in the class was looking at me and they were about to laugh.	○	○	○	○	○

14. *You invite a friend to sleep over. But when you ask your mother she says no.*

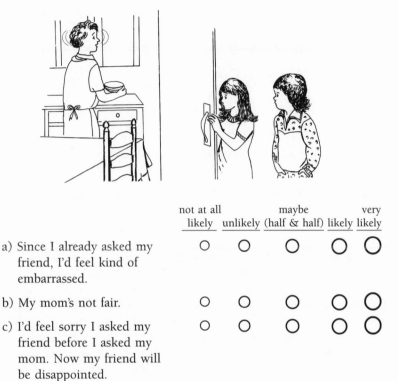

	not at all likely	unlikely	maybe (half & half)	likely	very likely
a) Since I already asked my friend, I'd feel kind of embarrassed.	O	O	O	O	O
b) My mom's not fair.	O	O	O	O	O
c) I'd feel sorry I asked my friend before I asked my mom. Now my friend will be disappointed.	O	O	O	O	O
d) My friend can always sleep over another time.	O	O	O	O	O

15. *Your teacher picks one student to do something special. She picks you.*

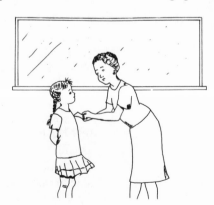

	not at all likely	unlikely	maybe (half & half)	likely	very likely
a) I'd be wondering how the other students felt—the ones that didn't get picked.	O	O	O	O	O
b) My friends will think I'm a teacher's pet.	O	O	O	O	O
c) I must have done a good job to have the teacher pick me.	O	O	O	O	O
d) I'd feel good about myself, like I'm special.	O	O	O	O	O
e) The teacher must really like me.	O	O	O	O	O

We are now recommending the use of the TOSCA-C in place of the SCAAI-C. The TOSCA-C is composed of 10 negative and 5 positive scenarios yielding indices of Shame-Proneness, Guilt-Proneness, Externalization, Detachment/Unconcern, Alpha Pride, and Beta Pride. The new scenarios were drawn from written accounts of personal shame, guilt, and pride experiences provided by a sample of about 140 children 8–12 years old. The new responses were drawn from a much larger pool of affective, cognitive, and behavioral responses provided by a second sample of 8–12 year olds. We are currently preparing a detailed report of two recent studies which supports the reliability and validity of the TOSCA-C.

The TOSCA-C has several advantages over the original SCAAI-C. The items were "subject generated" rather than "experimenter generated." And preliminary analyses indicate that the TOSCA-C is more psychometrically sound than the SCAAI-C.

Scoring for the TOSCA-C*:

1. a) Guilt
   b) Externalization
   c) Shame
   d) Alpha Pride
   e) Beta Pride
2. a) Guilt
   b) Detached
   c) Shame
   d) Externalization

9. a) Detached
   b) Externalization
   c) Shame
   d) Guilt
10. a) Externalization
    b) Detached
    c) Guilt
    d) Shame
11. a) Externalization

3. a) Guilt
   b) Shame
   c) Detached
   d) Externalization
4. a) Guilt
   b) Beta Pride
   c) Externalization
   d) Shame
   e) Alpha Pride
5. a) Detached
   b) Guilt
   c) Shame
   d) Externalization
6. a) Shame
   b) Guilt
   c) Detached
   d) Externalization
7. a) Externalization
   b) Shame
   c) Beta Pride
   d) Alpha Pride
   e) Guilt
8. a) Guilt
   b) Shame
   c) Detached
   d) Externalization

   b) Shame
   c) Guilt
   d) Detached
12. a) Externalization
   b) Guilt
   c) Alpha Pride
   d) Beta Pride
   e) Shame
13. a) Guilt
   b) Detached
   c) Externalization
   d) Shame
14. a) Shame
   b) Externalization
   c) Guilt
   d) Detached
15. a) Guilt
   b) Shame
   c) Beta Pride
   d) Alpha Pride
   e) Externalization

---

*Scale scores are the sum of responses to relevant items (e.g., the score for the Shame scale equals the respondent's answer to 1c, plus the answer to 2c, plus the answer to 3b, etc.).

SUBSCALE MEANS AND STANDARD DEVIATIONS FOR TOSCA-3, TOSCA-A, AND TOSCA-C

TOSCA-3: Subscale Means and Standard Deviations

Sample description	Sex	Shame	Guilt	Externalization	Detachment	Alpha Pride	Beta Pride
TOSCA-3: Students from a large public university enrolled in psychology courses (MAL9596)	Female (n = 142)	44.93 (11.32)	63.43 (7.51)	37.21 (8.44)	31.80 (6.42)	19.14 (3.42)	19.65 (3.27)
	Male (N = 45)	40.58 (10.36)	59.95 (7.49)	37.33 (8.09)	32.53 (5.86)	18.87 (2.79)	19.38 (2.77)
TOSCA-3: Students from a large public university enrolled in psychology courses (First impressions)	Female (n = 275)	45.49 (9.49)	64.09 (6.54)	37.83 (7.55)	31.41 (5.95)	20.44 (2.74)	20.96 (2.78)
	Male (n = 104)	40.93 (8.44)	59.57 (7.15)	38.28 (8.47)	32.27 (5.03)	19.74 (2.42)	20.63 (2.65)
TOSCA-3: Students from a large public university enrolled in psychology courses (Forgiveness-2)	Female (n = 217)	48.33 (9.32)	65.43 (7.54)	38.05 (8.78)	31.18 (6.78)	20.19 (2.92)	20.55 (2.88)
	Male (n = 51)	42.88 (10.15)	61.33 (7.54)	42.18 (10.09)	34.87 (6.71)	20.68 (2.89)	20.51 (2.98)

Note. Standard deviations appear in parentheses below means. Shame, Guilt, and Externalization scales are derived from 16 items each, Detachment from 11 items, and Alpha Pride and Beta Pride from 5 items each. Items are rated on a 5-point scale (1–5). These samples were fairly diverse in terms of age, socioeconomic status, and ethnic background owing to the relatively high proportion of commuter and returning students at this institution.

Child and Adolescent Versions: The TOSCA-C and TOSCA-A Subscale Means and Standard Deviations

Sample description	Sex	Shame	Guilt	Externalization	Detachment	Alpha Pride	Beta Pride
TOSCA-C: 5th-grade children from an ethnically and socioeconomically diverse urban public school system (IG90)	Female (n = 204)	42.78 (9.61)	60.18 (7.39)	40.63 (7.67)	28.68 (5.53)	18.88 (3.29)	19.68 (2.72)
	Male (n = 176)	39.97 (9.76)	56.06 (9.97)	43.69 (8.28)	30.43 (5.50)	18.83 (3.33)	19.56 (3.14)
TOSCA-C: 4th, 5th, and 6th graders from an ethnically and socioeconomically diverse public school system (PGKID91)	Female (n = 158)	43.06 (8.47)	58.51 (8.50)	42.97 (7.66)	31.04 (5.30)	19.38 (3.28)	19.99 (2.83)
	Male (n = 153)	38.80 (9.80)	54.59 (10.90)	43.41 (8.01)	31.60 (5.47)	19.09 (3.76)	20.05 (3.20)
TOSCA-A: Students in grades 7–11 from an ethnically and socioeconomically diverse urban public school system (PGADOL91)	Female (n = 230)	38.16 (8.55)	57.33 (7.92)	35.24 (8.05)	30.78 (5.11)	18.60 (2.94)	20.05 (2.55)
	Male (n = 209)	36.37 (8.54)	51.48 (8.95)	40.39 (8.82)	32.45 (5.18)	18.43 (3.30)	19.41 (2.90)
TOSCA-A: 7th-grade children from an ethnically and socioeconomically diverse urban public school system (IG92)	Female (n = 139)	37.82 (8.08)	58.09 (7.77)	37.51 (9.46)	31.31 (6.01)	18.62 (2.85)	19.85 (3.00)
	Male (n = 112)	37.09 (8.04)	52.17 (8.83)	40.63 (8.15)	32.23 (4.41)	18.14 (2.87)	19.05 (2.70)
TOSCA-A: College students from a large public university receiving credit for a psychology course requirement (MAL9596)	Female (n = 234)	39.82 (8.76)	60.05 (6.41)	35.21 (7.11)	30.86 (4.83)	18.46 (2.80)	20.32 (2.50)
	Male (n = 138)	37.97 (8.77)	57.47 (6.81)	36.50 (7.44)	31.09 (4.81)	18.04 (2.92)	19.48 (2.65)
TOSCA-A: Late adolescents (18–21 years) from an ethnically and socioeconomically diverse urban area (IG97)	Female (n = 152)	34.74 (8.38)	59.05 (6.65)	33.71 (6.51)	30.95 (5.10)	19.01 (2.57)	20.61 (2.33)
	Male (n = 117)	32.94 (6.98)	54.88 (8.18)	35.25 (6.23)	32.38 (4.52)	18.75 (2.54)	19.81 (2.02)

Note. Standard deviations appear in parentheses below means. Shame, Guilt, and Externalization scales are derived from 15 items each, Detachment from 10 items, and Alpha Pride and Beta Pride from 5 items each. Items are rated on a 5-point scale (1–5).

Reliabilities (Cronbach's Alpha) for the TOSCA-C, TOSCA-A, and TOSCA-3

Sample	n	Shame	Guilt	Externalization	Detachment	Alpha Pride	Beta Pride
TOSCA-C							
IG90	380	.78	.79	.66	.55	.47	.34
PGKID91	324	.78	.83	.64	.53	.58	.47
TOSCA-A							
PGADOL91	439	.77	.81	.76	.56	.51	.43
IG92	251	.79	.84	.82	.67	.44	.53
MAL9596	368–372	.84	.77	.78	.61	.49	.53
IG97	271	.82	.82	.71	.66	.49	.50
TOSCA-3							
MAL9596	184–187	.88	.83	.80	.77	.72	.72
First Impressions	368–376	.76	.70	.66	.60	.41	.55
Forgiveness-2	260–265	.77	.78	.75	.72	.48	.51

Note. For the TOSCA-A and TOSCA-C, Shame, Guilt, and Externalization scales are derived from 15 items each, Detachment from 10 items, and Alpha Pride and Beta Pride from 5 items each. For the TOSCA-3, Shame, Guilt, and Externalization scales are derived from 16 items each, Detachment from 11 items, and Alpha Pride and Beta Pride from 5 items each. In all versions, items are rated on a 5-point scale (1–5).

STATE SHAME AND GUILT SCALE (SSGS)

The following are some statements which may or may not describe how you are feeling *right now*. Please rate each statement using the 5-point scale below. Remember to rate each statement based on how you are feeling *right at this moment*.

	Not feeling this way at all	Feeling this way somewhat	Feeling this way very strongly

1. I feel good about myself. 1 - - - - 2 - - - - 3 - - - - 4 - - - -5

2. I want to sink into the floor and disappear. 1 - - - - 2 - - - - 3 - - - - 4 - - - -5

3. I feel remorse, regret. 1 - - - - 2 - - - - 3 - - - - 4 - - - -5

4. I feel worthwhile, valuable. 1 - - - - 2 - - - - 3 - - - - 4 - - - -5

5. I feel small. 1 - - - - 2 - - - - 3 - - - - 4 - - - -5

6. I feel tension about something I have done. 1 - - - - 2 - - - - 3 - - - - 4 - - - -5

7. I feel capable, useful. 1 - - - - 2 - - - - 3 - - - - 4 - - - -5

8. I feel like I am a bad person. 1 - - - - 2 - - - - 3 - - - - 4 - - - -5

9. I cannot stop thinking about something bad I have done. 1 - - - - 2 - - - - 3 - - - - 4 - - - -5

10. I feel proud. 1 - - - - 2 - - - - 3 - - - - 4 - - - -5

11. I feel humiliated, disgraced. 1 - - - - 2 - - - - 3 - - - - 4 - - - -5

12. I feel like apologizing, confessing. 1 - - - - 2 - - - - 3 - - - - 4 - - - -5

13. I feel pleased about something I have done. 1 - - - - 2 - - - - 3 - - - - 4 - - - -5

14. I feel worthless, powerless. 1 - - - - 2 - - - - 3 - - - - 4 - - - -5

15. I feel bad about something I have done. 1 - - - - 2 - - - - 3 - - - - 4 - - - -5

The SSGS is a self-rating scale of in-the-moment (state) feelings of shame, guilt, and pride experiences. Fifteen items (five for each of the three subscales) are rated on a 5-point Likert scale.

Examples of shame items include: "I want to sink into the floor and disappear," and "I feel small." Examples of guilt items include "I feel remorse, regret," and "I feel like apologizing, confessing." Examples of pride items include "I feel good about myself," and "I feel capable, useful."

The SSGS was initially developed as a manipulation check for the shame induction in an experimental study of shame and empathy (Marschall, 1996). The items for each subscale were derived from the empirical and theoretical literature. Participants were asked to complete the questionnaire as a "mood check," immediately following the shame induction.

The sample was drawn from a large east coast university population. Students were enrolled in an introductory psychology class and were offered credit for their participation. The students ranged in age from 17 to 42 ($M = 21.1$) and 69% were female; 70% were white, 9% black, 11% Asian, 4% Hispanic, and 8% other.

Results were as follows:

Scale	Mean sum (SD) (control participants) ($n = 82$)	Mean sum (SD) (induced shame participants) ($n = 60$)	Interitem reliability (all participants) ($n = 142$)
Shame	6.71 (2.60)	7.81 (4.01)	.89
Guilt	7.39 (2.87)	8.37 (3.84)	.82
Pride	16.83 (4.05)	15.90 (4.90)	.87

Participants reported higher levels of shame following the shame induction, as compared to nonshamed control participants ($t = -1.89, p < .05$). Participants who were shamed also reported greater levels of guilt than did control participants ($t = -1.69, p < .05$).

Scoring for the SSGS:

Each scale consists of 5 items:

- Shame—Items 2, 5, 8, 11, 14
- Guilt—Items 3, 6, 9, 12, 15
- Pride—Items 1, 4, 7, 10, 13

All items are scored in a positive direction.

REFERENCES

Abell, E., & Gecas, V. (1997). Guilt, shame, and family socialization: A retrospective study. *Journal of Family Issues, 18*, 99–123.

Abramson, L. Y., Seligman, M. E. P., & Teasdale, J. (1978). Learned helplessness in humans: Critique and reformulation. *Journal of Abnormal Psychology, 87*, 49–74.

Achenbach, T. M., & Edelbrock, C. (1986). *Manual for the teacher's report form and teacher version of the Child Behavior Profile*. Burlington: University of Vermont, Department of Psychiatry.

Alessandri, S., & Lewis, M. (1993). Parental evaluation and its relation to shame and pride in young children. *Sex Roles, 29*, 335–343.

Alessandri, S., & Lewis, M. (1996). Differences in pride and shame in maltreated and nonmaltreated preschoolers. *Child Development, 67*, 1857–1869.

Allan, S., Gilbert, P., & Goss, K. (1994). An exploration of shame measures. II: Psychopathology. *Personality and Individual Differences, 17*, 719–722.

American Psychiatric Association. (1994). *Diagnostic and statistical manual of mental disorders* (4th ed.). Washington, DC: Author.

Amsterdam, B. (1972). Mirror self-image reactions before age two. *Developmental Psychobiology, 5*, 297–305.

Andrews, B. (1995). Bodily shame as a mediator between abusive experiences and depression. *Journal of Abnormal Psychology, 104*, 277–285.

Andrews, B. (1998). Shame and childhood abuse. In P. Gilbert & B. Andrews (Eds.), *Shame: Interpersonal behavior, psychopathology, and culture* (pp. 176–190). New York: Oxford University Press.

Andrews, B., & Hunter, E. (1997). Shame, early abuse and course of depression in a clinical sample: A preliminary study. *Cognition and Emotions, 11*, 373–381.

Andrews, B., Qian, M., & Valentine, J. D. (in press). The role of shame in the prediction of depressive symptoms. *British Journal of Clinical Psychology*.

Andrews, D. A., & Bonta, J. (1994). *The psychology of criminal conduct*. Cincinnati, OH: Anderson.

Arnold, M. L. (1989). *Moral cognition and conduct: A qualitative review of the literature.*

Poster presented at the annual meeting of the Society for Research in Child Development, Kansas City, MO.

Arora, J. M. (1998). *Implications of characterological vs. behavioral self-blame for adjustment to negative life events*. Unpublished doctoral dissertation, George Mason University, Fairfax, VA.

Averill, J. R. (1982). *Anger and aggression: An essay on emotion*. New York: Springer-Verlag.

Barrett, K. C. (1995). A functionalist approach to shame and guilt. In J. P. Tangney & K. W. Fischer (Eds.), *Self-conscious emotions: The psychology of shame, guilt, embarrassment, and pride* (pp. 25–63). New York: Guilford Press.

Barrett, K. C., Ferguson, T. J., Smith, A. M., & Bertuzzi, J. S. (2000, April). *Adaptive shame and maladaptive pride in children and young adults: Insights from narratives of actual emotion episodes*. Poster presented at the Conference on Human Development, Memphis, TN.

Barrett, K. C., Zahn-Waxler, C., & Cole, P. M. (1993). Avoiders versus amenders: Implications for the investigation of shame and guilt during toddlerhood? *Cognition and Emotion, 7*, 481–505.

Batson, C. D. (1990). How social an animal? The human capacity for caring. *American Psychologist, 45*, 336–346.

Batson, C. D., & Coke, J. S. (1981). Empathy: A source of altruistic motivation for helping? In J. P. Rushton & R. M. Sorrentino (Eds.), *Altruism and helping behavior: Social, personality, and developmental perspectives* (pp. 167–187). Hillsdale, NJ: Erlbaum.

Batson, C. D., Dyck, J. L., Brandt, J. R., Batson, J. G., Powell, A. L., McMaster, M. R., & Griffitt, C. (1988). Five studies testing two new egoistic alternatives to the empathy–altruism hypothesis. *Journal of Personality and Social Psychology, 55*, 52–77.

Baumeister, R. F., Stillwell, A. M., & Heatherton, T. F. (1994). Guilt: An interpersonal approach. *Psychological Bulletin, 115*, 243–267.

Baumeister, R. F., Stillwell, A. M., & Heatherton, T. F. (1995). Interpersonal aspects of guilt: Evidence from narrative studies. In J. P. Tangney & K. W. Fischer (Eds.), *Self-conscious emotions: The psychology of shame, guilt, embarrassment, and pride* (pp. 255–273). New York: Guilford Press.

Baumrind, D. (1967). Child care practices anteceding three patterns of preschool behavior. *Genetic Psychology Monographs, 75*, 43–88.

Baumrind, D. (1971). Current patterns of parental authority. *Developmental Psychology, 4*, 1–103.

Baumrind, D. (1986). Sex differences in the development of moral reasoning: Response to Walker's (1984) conclusion that there are none. *Child Development, 57*, 511–521.

Beall, L. (1972). *Shame–Guilt Test*. Berkeley, CA: Wright Institute.

Beck, A. T. (1983). Cognitive therapy of depression: New perspectives. In P. Clayton & J. Barrett (Eds.), *Treatment of depression: Old controversies and new approaches* (pp. 265–290). New York: Raven Press.

Belsky, J., Woodworth, S., & Crnic, K. (1996). Troubled family interaction during toddlerhood. *Development & Psychopathology, 8*, 477–495.

Benedict, R. (1946). *The chrysanthemum and the sword*. Boston: Houghton Mifflin.

Benoit, D., & Parker, K. C. H. (1994). Stability and transmission of attachment across three generations. *Child Development, 65*, 1444–1456.

Berkowitz, L. (1962). *Aggression: A social psychological analysis*. New York: McGraw-Hill.

Berkowitz, L. (1969). *Roots of aggression: A re-examination of the frustration–aggression hypothesis*. New York: Atherton Press.

Berkowitz, L. (1993). *Aggression: Its causes, consequences, and control.* Philadelphia: Temple University Press.

Bertenthal, B. L., & Fischer, K. W. (1978). Development of self-recognition in the infant. *Developmental Psychology, 14,* 44–50.

Binder, J. L. (1970). The relative proneness to shame or guilt as a dimension of character style. *Dissertation Abstracts International, 32,* 1833B.

Blackburn, R. (1993). *The psychology of criminal conduct.* Chichester, UK: Wiley.

Blasi, A. (1980). Bridging moral cognition and moral action: A critical review of the literature. *Psychological Bulletin, 88,* 1–45.

Blatt, S. (1974). Levels of object representation in anaclitic and introjective depression. *Psychoanalytic Study of the Child, 29,* 107–157.

Block, J. H., Block, J., & Morrison, A. (1981). Parental agreement–disagreement on child-rearing orientations and gender-related personality correlates in children. *Child Development, 52,* 965–974.

Borenstein, J. K., & Tangney, J. P. (2001). *Cognitive and affective factors associated with HIV-related health knowledge and behaviors: Shame, blame, and depression.* Manuscript under review.

Bradshaw, J. (1988). *Healing the shame that binds you.* Deerfield Beach, FL: Health Communications.

Braithwaite, J. (1989). *Crime, shame, and reintegration.* Cambridge, UK: Cambridge University Press.

Braithwaite, J., & Mugsford, S. (1994). Conditions of successful reintegration ceremonies. *British Journal of Criminology, 34,* 139–171.

Brodie, P. (1995). *How sociopaths love: Sociopathy and interpersonal relationships.* Unpublished doctoral dissertation, George Mason University, Fairfax, VA.

Brown, H. N. (1987). The impact of suicide on therapists in training. *Comprehensive Psychiatry, 28,* 101–112.

Burggraf, S. A., & Tangney, J. P. (1989). *The Self-Conscious Affect and Attribution Inventory for Children (SCAAI-C).* Bryn Mawr College, Bryn Mawr, PA.

Burggraf, S. A., & Tangney, J. P. (1990). *Shame-proneness, guilt-proneness, and attributional style related to children's depression.* Poster presented at the annual meeting of the American Psychological Society, Dallas, TX.

Buss, A. H., & Durkee, A. (1957). An inventory for assessing different kinds of hostility in clinical situations. *Journal of Consulting Psychology, 21,* 343–348.

Buss, D. M., & Scheir, M. F. (1976). Self-consciousness, self-awareness, and self-attribution. *Journal of Research in Personality, 10,* 463–468.

Bybee, J., & Tangney, J. P. (Chairs). (1996). *Is guilt adaptive?: Functions in interpersonal relationships and mental health.* Symposium presented at the annual meeting of the American Psychological Association, Toronto, Ontario, Canada.

Cashdan, S. (1988). *Object relations therapy: Using the relationship.* New York: Norton.

Chandler-Holtz, D. M. (1999). Relations between negative self-conscious emotions and prosocial behavior, psychological functioning, and perceived parenting among adolescents. *Dissertation Abstracts International: Section B. The Sciences and Engineering, 60,* 1341.

Cheek, J. M., & Hogan, R. (1983). Self-concepts, self-presentations, and moral judgments. In J. Suls & A. G. Greenwald (Eds.), *Psychological perspectives on the self* (Vol. 2, pp. 249–273). Hillsdale, NJ: Erlbaum.

Chemtob, C. M., Hamada, R. S., Bauer, G., Kinney, B., & Torigoe, M. (1988). Patients' suicides: Frequency and impact on psychiatrists. *American Journal of Psychiatry, 145,* 224–228.

Christensen, A., Margolin, G., & Sullaway, M. (1992). Interparental agreement on child behavior problems. *Psychological Assessment, 4,* 419–425.

Cochran, S., & Mays, V. (1990). Sex, lies, and HIV. *New England Journal of Medicine, 11*, 774–775.

Coke, J. S., Batson, C. D., & McDavis, K. (1978). Empathic mediation of helping: A two-stage model. *Journal of Personality and Social Psychology, 36*, 752–766.

Cook, D. R. (1988). *The measurement of shame: The Internalized Shame Scale.* Paper presented at the annual meeting of the American Psychological Association, Atlanta, GA.

Cook, D. R. (1989). *Internalized Shame Scale (ISS).* University of Wisconsin, Stout.

Cook, D. R. (1991). Shame, attachment, and addictions: Implications for family therapists. *Contemporary Family Therapy, 13*, 405–419.

Coopersmith, S. (1967). *The antecedents of self-esteem.* San Francisco: Freeman.

Covert, M. V. (2000). *Effects of experimentally-induced shame on indirect aggression.* Unpublished doctoral dissertation (in progress), George Mason University, Fairfax, VA.

Crouppen, G. A. (1976). Field dependence–independence in depressive and "normal" males as an indicator of relative proneness to shame or guilt and ego-functioning. *Dissertation Abstracts International, 37*, 4669B-4670B.

Damon, W. (1988). *The moral child: Nurturing children's natural moral growth.* New York: Free Press.

Damon, W., & Hart, D. (1982). Development of self-understanding from infancy through adolescence. *Child Development, 53*, 841–864.

Darvill, T. J., Johnson, R. C., & Danko, G. P. (1992). Personality correlates of public and private self-consciousness. *Personality and Individual Differences, 13*, 383–384.

Davis, D., & Brock, T. C. (1975). Use of first person pronouns as a function of increased objective self-awareness and performance feedback. *Journal of Experimental Social Psychology, 11*, 381–388.

Davis, M. H. (1980). A multidimensional approach to individual differences in empathy. *JSAS Catalog of Selected Documents in Psychology, 10*, 85.

Davis, M. H. (1983). Measuring individual differences in empathy: Evidence for a multidimensional approach. *Journal of Personality and Social Psychology, 44*, 113–126.

Davis, M. H., & Oathout, H. A. (1987). Maintenance of satisfaction in romantic relationships: Empathy and relational competence. *Journal of Personality and Social Psychology, 53*, 397–410.

Dekovic, M., & Janssens, J. M. A. M. (1992). Parents' child-rearing style and children's sociometric status. *Developmental Psychology, 28*, 925–932.

Denham, S. A., & Couchoud, E. A. (1991). Social-emotional predictors of preschoolers' responses to adult negative emotion. *Journal of Child Psychology and Psychiatry, 32*, 595–608.

Derogatis, L. R., Lipman, R. S., & Covi, L. (1973). The SCL-90: An outpatient psychiatric rating scale. *Psychopharmacology Bulletin, 9*, 13–28.

Diamond, M. (1993). Homosexuality and bisexuality in different populations. *Archives of Sexual Behavior, 22*, 291–310.

Dix, T. (1991). The affective organization of parenting: Adaptive and maladaptive processes. *Psychological Bulletin, 110*, 3–25.

Durkheim, E. (1966). *Suicide: A study in sociology.* New York: Free Press.

Dutton, D. G. (1995). Male abusiveness in intimate relationships. *Clinical Psychology Review, 15*, 567–581.

Dutton, D. G. (1998). *The abusive personality.* New York: Guilford Press.

Dutton, D. G. (1999). Traumatic origins of intimate rage. *Aggression and Violent Behavior, 4*, 431–447.

Dutton, D. G., van Ginkel, C., & Starzomski, A. (1995). The role of shame and guilt in the intergenerational transmission of abusiveness. *Violence and Victims, 10*, 121–131.

Duval, S., & Wicklund, R. A. (1972). *A theory of objective self-awareness.* New York: Academic Press.

Duval, S., & Wicklund, R. A. (1973). Effects of objective self-awareness on attribution of causality. *Journal of Experimental Social Psychology, 9*, 17–31.

Dweck, C. S., Hong, Y., & Chiu, C. (1993). Implicit theories: Individual differences in the likelihood and meaning of dispositional inferences. *Personality and Social Psychology Bulletin, 19*, 644–656.

Dweck, C. S., & Leggett, E. L. (1988). A social-cognitive approach to motivation and personality. *Psychological Review, 95*, 256–273.

Eisenberg, N. (1986). *Altruistic cognition, emotion, and behavior.* Hillsdale, NJ: Erlbaum.

Eisenberg, N. (2000). Motion, regulation, and moral development. *Annual Review of Psychology, 51*, 665–697.

Eisenberg, N., Fabes, R. A., Carlo, G., Speer, A. L., Switzer, G., Karbon, M., & Troyer, D. (1993). The relations of empathy-related emotions and maternal practices to children's comforting behavior. *Journal of Experimental Child Psychology, 55*, 131–150.

Eisenberg, N., Fabes, R. A., Miller, P. A., Shell, R., Shea, C., & Mayplumlee, T. (1990). Pre-schoolers' vicarious emotional responding and their situational and dispositional prosocial behavior. *Merrill-Palmer Quarterly, 36*, 507–529.

Eisenberg, N., Fabes, R. A., Murphy, B., Karbon, M., Smith, M., & Maszk, P. (1996). The relations of children's dispositional empathy-related responding to their emotionality, regulation, and social functioning. *Developmental Psychology, 32*, 195–209.

Eisenberg, N., Fabes, R., & Shea, C. (1989). Gender differences in empathy and prosocial moral reasoning: Empirical investigations. In M. M. Brabeck (Ed.), *Who cares?: Theory, research, and educational implications of the ethic of care* (pp. 127–143). New York: Praeger.

Eisenberg, N., & Miller, P. A. (1987). Empathy, sympathy and altruism: Empirical and conceptual links. In N. Eisenberg & J. Strayer (Eds.), *Empathy and its development* (pp. 292–311). New York: Cambridge University Press.

Eisenberg-Berg, N., & Neal, C. (1979). Children's moral reasoning about their own spontaneous prosocial behavior. *Developmental Psychology, 15*, 228–229.

Ekman, P., Friesen, W. V., & Ellsworth, P. C. (1982). What are the similarities and differences in facial behavior across cultures? In P. Ekman (Ed.), *Emotion in the human face* (pp. 128–143). Cambridge, UK: Cambridge University Press.

Ellis, A. (1962). *Reason and emotion in psychotherapy.* New York: Stuart.

Emmons, R. A. (1984). Factor analysis and construct validity of the Narcissistic Personality Inventory. *Journal of Personality Assessment, 48*, 291–300.

Epstein, S. (1980). The self-concept: A review and the proposal of an integrated theory of personality. In E. Staub (Ed.), *Personality: Basic aspects and current research* (pp. 82–132). Englewood Cliffs, NJ: Prentice-Hall.

Erikson, E. H. (1950). *Childhood and society.* New York: Norton.

Estrada, P. (1995). Adolescents' self-reports of prosocial responses to friends and acquaintances: The role of sympathy-related cognitive, affective, and motivational processes. *Journal of Research on Adolescence, 5*, 173–200.

Exner, J. E., Jr. (1986). *The Rorschach: A comprehensive system* (Vol. 1). New York: Wiley.

Fee, R. L. (1998). [Help-seeking behaviors among clinical psychology graduate students in the Washington, DC, metropolitan area.] Unpublished raw data, George Mason University, Fairfax, VA.

Fenigstein, A., Scheier, M. F., & Buss, A. H. (1975). Public and private self-consciousness: Assessment and theory. *Journal of Consulting and Clinical Psychology, 43,* 522–527.

Ferguson, T. J., Barrett, K. C., Edmondson, R. S., Eyre, H. L., Ashbaker, M., Grotepas-Sanders, D., Van Wagoner, R., & Hawkins, S. (2000, February). *Adaptive and maladaptive features of shame.* Paper presented at the annual meeting of the Society for Personality and Social Psychology, Nashville, TN.

Ferguson, T. J., & Eyre, H. L. (2001). *Reconciling interpersonal versus appraisal views of guilt: Roles of inductive strategies and projected responsibility in prolonging guilty feelings.* Manuscript under review.

Ferguson, T. J., & Rule, B. G. (1983). An attributional perspective on anger and aggression. In R. Geen & E. Donnerstein (Eds.), *Aggression: Theoretical and empirical reviews* (Vol. 1, pp. 41–74). New York: Academic Press.

Ferguson, T. J., & Stegge, H. (1995). Emotional states and traits in children: The case of guilt and shame. In J. P. Tangney & K. W. Fischer (Eds.), *Self-conscious emotions: The psychology of shame, guilt, embarrassment, and pride* (pp. 174–197). New York: Guilford Press.

Ferguson, T. J., Stegge, H., & Damhuis, I. (1990a). Guilt and shame experiences in elementary school-age children. In R. J. Takens (Ed.), *European perspectives in psychology* (Vol. 1, pp. 195–218). New York: Wiley.

Ferguson, T. J., Stegge, H., & Damhuis, I. (1990b). *Spontaneous and elicited guilt and shame experiences in elementary school-age children.* Poster presented at the annual meeting of the Southwestern Society for Research in Human Development, Dallas, TX.

Ferguson, T. J., Stegge, H., & Damhuis, I. (1991). Children's understanding of guilt and shame. *Child Development, 62,* 827–839.

Ferguson, T. J., Stegge, H., Miller, E. R., & Olsen, M. E. (1999). Guilt, shame, and symptoms in children. *Developmental Psychology, 35,* 347–357.

Feshbach, N. D. (1975a). Empathy in children: Some theoretical and empirical considerations. *Counseling Psychologist, 5,* 25–30.

Feshbach, N. D. (1975b). The relationship of child-rearing factors to children's aggression, empathy, and related positive and negative behaviors. In J. deWit & W. W. Hartup (Eds.), *Determinants and origins of aggressive behavior.* The Hague, Netherlands: Mouton.

Feshbach, N. D. (1978). Studies of empathic behavior in children. In B. A. Maher (Ed.), *Progress in experimental personality research* (Vol. 8, pp. 1–47). New York: Academic Press.

Feshbach, N. D. (1984). Empathy, empathy training, and the regulation of aggression in elementary school children. In R. M. Kaplan, V. J. Konenci, & R. Novoco (Eds.), *Aggression in children and youth.* The Hague, Netherlands: Nijhoff.

Feshbach, N. D. (1987). Parental empathy and child adjustment/maladjustment. In N. Eisenberg & J. Strayer (Eds.), *Empathy and its development* (pp. 271–291). New York: Cambridge University Press.

Feshbach, N. D., & Caskey, N. (1987). *Feshbach Parent/Partner Empathy Scale.* University of California, Los Angeles.

Feshbach, N. D., & Feshbach, S. (1969). The relationship between empathy and aggression in two age groups. *Developmental Psychology, 1,* 102–107.

Feshbach, N. D., & Feshbach, S. (1982). Empathy training and the regulation of aggression: Potentialities and limitations. *Academic Psychology Bulletin, 4,* 399–413.

Feshbach, N. D., & Feshbach, S. (1986). Aggression and altruism: A personality perspective. In C. Zahn-Waxler, E. M. Cummings, & R. Iannotti (Eds.), *Altruism and aggression: Biological and social origins* (pp. 189–217). Cambridge, UK: Cambridge University Press.

Feshbach, N. D., & Lipian, M. (1987). *The Empathy Scale for Adults*. Los Angeles: University of California, Los Angeles.

Fessler, D. M. T. (1999). Toward an understanding of the universality of second order emotions. In A. L. Hinton (Ed.), *Biocultural approaches to the emotions* (pp. 75–116). New York: Cambridge University Press.

Finch, A. J., Jr., Saylor, C. F., & Nelson, W. M., III. (1987). Assessment of anger in children. *Advances in Behavioral Assessment of Children and Families, 3,* 235–265.

Fischer, K. W., & Tangney, J. P. (1995). Self-conscious emotions and the affect revolution: Framework and overview. In J. P. Tangney & K. W. Fischer (Eds.), *Self-conscious emotions: The psychology of shame, guilt, embarrassment, and pride* (pp. 3–22). New York: Guilford Press.

Fitts, W. H. (1965). *Manual for the Tennessee Self Concept Scale*. Los Angeles: Western Psychological Services.

Fossum, M. A., & Mason, M. J. (1986). *Facing shame: Families in recovery*. New York: Norton.

Freud, S. (1953a). Further remarks on the neuro-psychoses of defence. In J. Strachey (Ed. & Trans.), *The standard edition of the complete psychological works of Sigmund Freud* (Vol. 3, pp. 157–185). London: Hogarth Press. (Original work published 1896)

Freud, S. (1953b). Three essays on the theory of sexuality. In J. Strachey (Ed. & Trans.), *The standard edition of the complete psychological works of Sigmund Freud* (Vol. 7, pp. 153–243). London: Hogarth Press. (Original work published 1905)

Freud, S. (1957). On narcissism: An introduction. In J. Strachey (Ed. & Trans.), *The standard edition of the complete psychological works of Sigmund Freud* (Vol. 14, pp. 73–102). London: Hogarth Press. (Original work published 1914)

Freud, S. (1961a). Civilization and its discontents. In J. Strachey (Ed. & Trans.), *The standard edition of the complete psychological works of Sigmund Freud* (Vol. 21, pp. 57–146). London: Hogarth Press. (Original work published 1930)

Freud, S. (1961b). Some psychical consequences of the anatomical distinction between the sexes. In J. Strachey (Ed. & Trans.), *The standard edition of the complete psychological works of Sigmund Freud* (Vol. 19, pp. 248–258). London: Hogarth Press. (Original work published 1925)

Freud, S. (1961c). The dissolution of the Oedipus Complex. In J. Strachey (Ed. & Trans.), *The standard edition of the complete psychological works of Sigmund Freud* (Vol. 19, pp. 173–182). London: Hogarth Press. (Original work published 1924)

Freud, S. (1961d). The id and the ego. In J. Strachey (Ed. & Trans.), *The standard edition of the complete psychological works of Sigmund Freud* (Vol. 19, pp. 12–66). London: Hogarth Press. (Original work published 1923)

Friedman, F. A. (1999). Correlations of shame and guilt to personality styles (MCMI—III). *Dissertation Abstracts International: Section B. The Sciences and Engineering, 60,* 3001.

Fultz, J., Batson, C. D., Fortenbach, V. A., McCarthy, P. M., & Varney, L. L. (1986). Social evaluation and the empathy-altruism hypothesis. *Journal of Personality and Social Psychology, 50,* 761–769.

Gehm, T. L., & Scherer, K. R. (1988). Relating situation evaluation to emotion differentiation: Nonmetric analysis of cross-cultural questionnaire data. In K. R. Scherer (Ed.), *Facets of emotion: Recent research* (pp. 61–77). Hillsdale, NJ: Erlbaum.

Gendreau, P., Little, T., & Goggin, C. (1996). A meta-analysis of the predictors of adult offender recidivism: What works. *Criminology, 34*, 575–607.

Gessner, T. L., & Tangney, J. P. (1990). *Personality and adjustment correlates of wit and witticism.* Poster presented at the annual meeting of the Eastern Psychological Association, Philadelphia, PA.

Gibbons, F. X., & Wicklund, R. A. (1982). Self-focused attention and helping behavior. *Journal of Personality and Social Psychology, 43*, 462–474.

Gilbert, P. (1997). The evolution of social attractivenenss and its role in shame, humiliation, guilt, and therapy. *British Journal of Medical Psychology, 70*, 113–147.

Gilbert, P., Allan, S., & Goss, K. (1996). Parental representations, shame, interpersonal problems, and vulnerability to psychopathology. *Clinical Psychology and Psychotherapy, 3*, 23–34.

Gilbert, P., & McGuire, M. T. (1998). Shame, status, and social roles: Psychobiology and evolution. In P. Gilbert & B. Andrews (Eds.), *Shame: Interpersonal behavior, psychopathology, and culture* (pp. 99–125). New York: Oxford University Press.

Gilbert, P., Pehl, J., & Allen, S. (1994). The phenomenology of shame and guilt: An empirical investigation. *British Journal of Medical Psychology, 67*, 23–36.

Gilligan, C. (1982). *In a different voice: Psychological theory and women's development.* Cambridge, MA: Harvard University Press.

Gilligan, C., & Attanucci, J. (1988). Two moral orientations: Gender differences and similarities. *Merrill–Palmer Quarterly, 34*, 223–237.

Gioiella, P. P. (1981). *The relationship of relative shame/guilt proneness to the attribution of responsibility under no shame and shame arousal.* Unpublished doctoral dissertation, New York University.

Goldberg, C. (1991). *Understanding shame.* Northvale, NJ: Aronson.

Gottman, J. M., & Declaire, J. (1998). *Raising an emotionally intelligent child.* New York: Simon & Schuster.

Gottschalk, L., & Gleser, G. (1969). *The measurement of psychological states through the content analysis of verbal behavior.* Berkeley: University of California Press.

Gramzow, R., & Tangney, J. P. (1992). Proneness to shame and the narcissistic personality. *Personality and Social Psychology Bulletin, 18*, 369–376.

Gray, J. (1992). *Men are from Mars, women are from Venus: A practical guide for improving communication and getting what you want in your relationships.* New York: HarperCollins.

Grusec, J. E., & Goodnow, J. J. (1994). Impact of parental discipline methods on the child's internalization of values: A reconceptualization of current points of view. *Developmental Psychology, 30*, 4–19.

Hanson, R. K., & Tangney, J. P. (1995). *The Test of Self-Conscious Affect–Socially Deviant Populations (TOSCA-SD).* Corrections Research, Department of the Solicitor General of Canada, Ottawa.

Harder, D. W. (1995). Shame and guilt assessment and relationships of shame and guilt proneness to psychopathology. In J. P. Tangney & K. W. Fischer (Eds.), *Self-conscious emotions: The psychology of shame, guilt, embarrassment, and pride* (pp. 368–392). New York: Guilford Press.

Harder, D. W., Cutler, L., & Rockart, L. (1992). Assessment of shame and guilt and their relationship to psychopathology. *Journal of Personality Assessment, 59*, 584–604.

Harder, D. W., & Lewis, S. J. (1987). The assessment of shame and guilt. In J. N. Butcher & C. D. Spielberger (Eds.), *Advances in personality assessment* (Vol. 6, pp. 89–114). Hillsdale, NJ: Erlbaum.

Harder, D. W., & Zalma, A. (1990). Two promising shame and guilt scales: A construct validity comparison. *Journal of Personality Assessment, 55*, 729–745.

Harris, G. T., Rice, M. E., & Quinsey, V. L. (1993). Violent recidivism of mentally disordered offenders: The development of a statistical prediction instrument. *Criminal Justice and Behavior, 20*, 315–335.

Harris, P. L. (1989). *Children and emotion: The development of psychological understanding.* New York: Blackwell.

Harris, P. L., Olthof, T., Terwogt, M. M., & Hardman, C. E. (1987). Children's knowledge of the situations that provoke emotion. *International Journal of Behavioral Development, 10*, 319–343.

Harter, S., & Whitesell, N. (1989). Developmental changes in children's emotion concepts. In C. Saarni & P. L. Harris (Eds.), *Children's understanding of emotions.* New York: Cambridge University Press.

Hartmann, E., & Loewenstein, R. (1962). Notes on the superego. *Psychoanalytic Study of the Child, 17*, 42–81.

Hassan, R. (1980). Suicide in Singapore. *European Journal of Sociology, 21*, 183–219.

Hassan, R. (1995). *Suicide explained.* Carlton South, Victoria, Australia: Melbourne University Press.

Hastings, M. E., Northman, L. M., & Tangney, J. P. (2000). Shame, guilt, and suicide. In T. E. Joiner & M. D. Rudd (Eds.), *Suicide science: Expanding the boundaries* (pp. 67–79). Norwell, MA: Kluwer.

Heider, F. (1958). *The psychology of interpersonal relations.* New York: Wiley.

Helgeson, V. S. (1994). Relation of agency and communion to well-being: Evidence and potential explanations. *Psychological Bulletin, 116*, 412–428.

Higgins, E. T. (1987). Self-discrepancy: A theory relating self and affect. *Psychological Review, 94*, 319–340.

Hoblitzelle, W. (1987a). Attempts to measure and differentiate shame and guilt: The relation between shame and depression. In H. B. Lewis (Ed.), *The role of shame in symptom formation* (pp. 207–235). Hillsdale, NJ: Erlbaum.

Hoblitzelle, W. (1987b). *The measurement of shame and guilt and the role of shame in depression.* Unpublished doctoral dissertation, Yale University, New Haven, CT.

Hoffman, M. L. (1970). Moral development. In P. H. Mussen (Ed.), *Carmichael's manual of child psychology* (Vol. 2, pp. 261–359). New York: Wiley.

Hoffman, M. L. (1982). Development of prosocial motivation: Empathy and guilt. In N. Eisenberg-Berg (Ed.), *Development of prosocial behavior* (pp. 281–313). New York: Academic Press.

Hoffman, M. L. (1984). Interaction of affect and cognition in empathy. In C. E. Izard, J. Kagan, & R. Zajonc (Eds.), *Emotion, cognition, and behavior* (pp. 103–131). Cambridge, UK: Cambridge University Press.

Hoffman, M. L. (1987). The contribution of empathy to justice and moral judgement. In N. Eisenberg & J. Strayer (Eds.), *Empathy and its development* (pp. 47–80). New York: Cambridge University Press.

Hoglund, C. L., & Nicholas, K. B. (1995). Shame, guilt, and anger in college students exposed to abusive family environments. *Journal of Family Violence, 10*, 141–157.

Holden, G. W., & Edwards, L. A. (1989). Parental attitudes toward child rearing: Instruments, issues, and implications. *Psychological Bulletin, 106*, 29–58.

Holtzworth-Munroe, A., & Hutchinson, G. (1993). Attributing negative intent to wife behavior: The attributions of maritally violent versus nonviolent men. *Journal of Abnormal Psychology, 102*, 206–211.

Huber, C. H., & Milstein, B. (1985). Cognitive restructuring and a collaborative set in couples work. *American Journal of Family Therapy, 13*, 17–27.

Huesmann, L. R., Eron, L. D., Lefkowitz, M. M., & Walder, L. O. (1984). Stability of aggression over time and generations. *Developmental Psychology, 20*, 1120–1134.

Ickes, W. J., Wicklund, R. A., & Ferris, C. B. (1973). Objective self awareness and self esteem. *Journal of Experimental Social Psychology, 9*, 202–219.

Indermaur, D. (1994). Offenders' perceptions of sentencing. *Australian Psychologist, 29*, 140–144.

Izard, C. E. (1977). *Human emotions.* New York: Plenum Press.

Jacobson, E. (1954). The self and the object world: Vicissitudes of their infantile cathexis and their influences on ideational and affective development. *Psychoanalytic Study of the Child, 9*, 75–127.

Jacoby, M. (1991). *Shame and the origins of self-esteem: A Jungian approach.* New York: Routledge.

Janoff-Bulman, R. (1979). Characterological versus behavioral self-blame: Inquiries into depression and rape. *Journal of Personality and Social Psychology, 37*, 1798–1809.

Johnson, R. C., Danko, G. P., Huang, Y. H., Park, J. Y., Johnson, S. B., & Nagoshi, C. T. (1987). Guilt, shame and adjustment in three cultures. *Personality and Individual Differences, 8*, 357–364.

Johnson, R. C., & Noel, R. (1970). *Dimensions of consciences.* Unpublished manuscript, University of Colorado, Boulder.

Jones, D. J., & Zelewski, C. (1994). Shame and depression proneness among female adult children of alcoholics. *International Journal of the Addictions, 29*, 1601–1609.

Jones, W. H., & Kugler, K. (1993). Interpersonal correlates of the Guilt Inventory. *Journal of Personality Assessment, 61*, 246–258.

Kahne, M. J. (1968). Suicide among patients in mental hospitals: A study of psychiatrists who conducted their psychotherapy. *Psychiatry, 31*, 32–43.

Karp, D. R. (1998). The judicial and judicious use of shame penalties. *Crime and Delinquency, 44*, 277–294.

Kaufman, G. (1985). *Shame: The power of caring.* Cambridge, MA: Schenkman.

Kaufman, G. (1989). *The psychology of shame: Theory and treatment of shame-based syndromes.* New York: Springer.

Kaufman, G., & Raphael, L. (1997). *Coming out of shame.* New York: Doubleday.

Keltner, D. (1995). Signs of appeasement: Evidence for the distinct displays of embarrassment, amusement, and shame. *Journal of Personality and Social Psychology, 68*, 441–454.

Keltner, D., & Buswell, B. N. (1996). Evidence for the distinctness of embarrassment, shame, and guilt: A study of recalled antecedents and facial expressions of emotion. *Cognition and Emotion, 10*, 155–171.

Keltner, D., & Harker, L. (1998). The forms and functions of the nonverbal signal of shame. In P. Gilbert & B. Andrews (Eds.), *Shame: Interpersonal behavior, psychopathology, and culture* (pp. 78–98). New York: Oxford University Press.

Kernberg, O. F. (1975). *Borderline conditions and pathological narcissism.* New York: Aronson.

Kernis, M. H., Grannemann, B. D., & Barclay, L. C. (1989). Stability and level of self-esteem as predictors of anger arousal and hostility. *Journal of Personality and Social Psychology, 56*, 1013–1022.

Kessler, B. L., & Bieschke, K. J. (1999). A retrospective analysis of shame, dissociation, and adult victimization in survivors of childhood sexual abuse. *Journal of Counseling Psychology, 46*, 335–341.

Klass, E. T. (1987). Situational approach to the assessment of guilt: Development and validation of a self-report measure. *Journal of Psychopathology and Behavioral Assessment, 9*, 35–48.

Kochanska, G. (1991). Socialization and temperament in the development of guilt and conscience. *Child Development, 62*, 1379–1392.

Kochanska, G. (1993). Toward a synthesis of parental socialization and child temperament in early development of conscience. *Child Development, 64*, 325–347.

Kochanska, G. (1994). Beyond cognition: Expanding the search for the early roots of internalization and conscience. *Developmental Psychology, 30*, 20–22.

Kohlberg, L. (1969). Stage and sequence: The cognitive developmental approach to socialization. In D. A. Goslin (Ed.), *Handbook of socialization theory and research* (pp. 347–480). Chicago: Rand McNally.

Kohut, H. (1971). *The analysis of the self.* New York: International Universities Press.

Kubany, E. S., Haynes, S. N., Abueg, F. R., Manke, F. P., Brennan, J. M., & Strahura, C. (1996). Development and validation of the Trauma-Related Guilt Inventory (TRGI). *Psychological Assessment, 8*, 428–444.

Kuczynski, L., Kochanska, G., Radke-Yarrow, M., & Girnius-Brown, O. (1987). A developmental interpretation of young children's noncompliance. *Developmental Psychology, 23*, 799–806.

Kugler, K., & Jones, W. H. (1992). On conceptualizing and assessing guilt. *Journal of Personality and Social Psychology, 62*, 318–327.

Kushner, M. G., & Sher, K. J. (1991). The relation of treatment fearfulness and psychological service utilization: An overview. *Professional Psychology: Research and Practice, 22*, 196–203.

Lansky, M. (1987). Shame and domestic violence. In D. L. Nathanson (Ed.), *The many faces of shame* (pp. 335–362) New York: Guilford Press.

Lansky, M. R., & Morrison, A. P. (1997). *The widening scope of shame.* Hillsdale, NJ: Analytic Press.

Leary, M. R. (1989, August). Fear of exclusion and appeasement behaviors: The case of blushing. In R. F. Baumeister (Chair), *The need to belong.* Symposium presented at the annual meeting of the American Psychological Association, New Orleans, LA.

Leary, M. R., Landel, J. L., & Patton, K. M. (1996). The motivated expression of embarrassment following a self-presentational predicament. *Journal of Personality, 64*, 619–637.

Leenaars, P. E., Rombouts, R., & Kok, G. (1993). Seeking medical care for a sexually transmitted disease: Determinants of delay-behavior. *Psychology and Health, 8*, 17–32.

Leith, K. P. (1998). Interpersonal conflict resolution: Guilt, shame, and counterfactual thinking. *Dissertation Abstracts International: Section B. The Sciences and Engineering, 58*, 5699.

Leith, K. P., & Baumeister, R. F. (1998). Empathy, shame, guilt, and narratives of interpersonal conflicts: Guilt-prone people are better at perspective taking. *Journal of Personality, 66*, 1–37.

Lester, D. (1998). The association of shame and guilt with suicidality. *Journal of Social Psychology, 138*, 535–536.

Lewis, H. B. (1971). *Shame and guilt in neurosis.* New York: International Universities Press.

Lewis, H. B. (1981). *Freud and modern psychology* (Vol. 1). New York: Plenum Press.

Lewis, H. B. (1987a). Introduction: Shame—the sleeper in psychopathology. In H. B. Lewis (Ed.), *The role of shame in symptom formation* (pp. 1–28). Hillsdale, NJ: Erlbaum.

Lewis, H. B. (1987b). Shame and the narcissistic personality. In D. L. Nathanson (Ed.), *The many faces of shame* (pp. 93–132). New York: Guilford Press.

Lewis, H. B. (1987c). The role of shame in depression over the life span. In H. B. Lewis (Ed.), *The role of shame in symptom formation* (pp. 29–50). Hillsdale, NJ: Erlbaum.

Lewis, H. B. (Ed.). (1987d). *The role of shame in symptom formation*. Hillsdale, NJ: Erlbaum.

Lewis, M. (1992). *Shame: The exposed self*. New York: Free Press.

Lewis, M., Alessandri, S., & Sullivan, M. W. (1992). Differences in shame and pride as a function of children's gender and task difficulty. *Child Development, 63*, 630–638.

Lewis, M., Sullivan, M. W., Stanger, C., & Weiss, M. (1989). Self-development and self-conscious emotions. *Child Development, 60*, 146–156.

Lindsay-Hartz, J. (1984). Contrasting experiences of shame and guilt. *American Behavioral Scientist, 27*, 689–704.

Lindsay-Hartz, J., de Rivera, J., & Mascolo, M. (1995). Differentiating shame and guilt and their effects on motivation. In J. P. Tangney & K. W. Fischer (Eds.), *Self-conscious emotions: The psychology of shame, guilt, embarrassment, and pride* (pp. 274–300). New York: Guilford Press.

Linehan, M. M. (1993a). *Skills training manual for treating borderline personality disorder*. New York: Guilford Press.

Linehan, M. M. (1993b). *Cognitive–behavioral treatment of borderline personality disorder*. New York: Guilford Press.

Lipian, M., & Feshbach, N. D. (1987). *Empathy Scale for Children*. University of California, Los Angeles.

Litman, R. (1965). When patients commit suicide. *American Journal of Psychotherapy, 19*, 570–576.

Lutwak, N., & Ferrari, J. R. (1997). Understanding shame in adults: Retrospective perceptions of parental-bonding during childhood. *Journal of Nervous and Mental Disease, 185*, 595–598.

Lytton, H. (1980). *Parent–child interaction: The socialization process observed in twin and singleton families*. New York: Plenum Press.

Maccoby, E. E., & Martin, J. A. (1983). Socialization in the context of the family: Parent–child interaction. In P. Mussen (Series Ed.) & E. M. Hetherington (Ed.), *Handbook of child psychology: Vol. 4. Socialization, personality, and social development* (4th ed., pp. 1–102). New York: Wiley.

Marks, G., Richardson, J. L., & Maldonado, N. (1991). Self-disclosure of HIV infection to sexual partners. *American Journal of Public Health, 81*, 1321–1322.

Marschall, D. E. (1996). *Effects of induced shame on subsequent empathy and altruistic behavior*. Unpublished master's thesis, George Mason University, Fairfax, VA.

Marschall, D., Sanftner, J., & Tangney, J. P. (1994). *The State Shame and Guilt Scale*. George Mason University, Fairfax, VA.

Mascolo, M. F., & Fischer, K. W. (1995). Developmental transformation in appraisals for pride, shame, and guilt. In J. P. Tangney & K. W. Fischer (Eds.), *Self-conscious emotions: The psychology of shame, guilt, embarrassment, and pride* (pp. 64–113). New York: Guilford Press.

Massaro, T. M. (1997). The meanings of shame: Implications for legal reform. *Psychology, Public Policy, and Law, 3*, 645–704.

Meehan, M. A., O'Connor, L. E., Berry, J. W., Weiss, J., Morrison, A., & Acampora, A. (1996). Guilt, shame, and depression in clients in recovery from addiction. *Journal of Psychoactive Drugs, 28*, 125–134.

Miller, P. A., & Eisenberg, N. (1988). The relation of empathy to aggressive and externalizing/antisocial behavior. *Psychological Bulletin, 103*, 324–344.

Miller, S. B. (1985). *The shame experience*. Hillsdale, NJ: Erlbaum.

Miller, S. B. (1996). *Shame in context*. Hillsdale, NJ: Analytic Press.

Mollon, R. (1984). Shame in relation to narcissistic disturbance. *British Journal of Medical Psychology, 57*, 207–214.

Morrison, A. P. (1983). Shame, ideal self, and narcissism. *Contemporary Psychoanalysis, 19,* 295–318.

Morrison, A. P. (1989). *Shame: The underside of narcissism.* Hillsdale, NJ: Analytic Press.

Morrison, A. P. (1996). *The culture of shame.* New York: Ballantine Books.

Morrison, N. K. (1987). The role of shame in schizophrenia. In H. B. Lewis (Ed.), *The role of shame in symptom formation* (pp. 51–87). Hillsdale, NJ: Erlbaum.

Mosher, D. L. (1966). The development and multitrait–multimethod matrix analysis of three measures of three aspects of guilt. *Journal of Consulting and Clinical Psychology, 30,* 25–29.

Mosher, D. L., & White, B. B. (1981). On differentiating shame and shyness. *Motivation and Emotion, 1,* 61–74.

Mugsford, J., & Mugsford, S. (1991). *Shame and reintegration in the punishment and deterrence of spousal abuse.* Paper presented at the American Society of Criminology Conference, San Francisco.

Mullins, L. S., & Kopelman, R. E. (1988). Toward an assessment of the construct validity of four measures of narcissism. *Journal of Personality Assessment, 52,* 610–625.

Nathanson, D. L. (1987a). A timetable for shame. In D. L. Nathanson (Ed.), *The many faces of shame* (pp. 1–63). New York: Guilford Press.

Nathanson, D. L. (Ed.). (1987b). *The many faces of shame.* New York: Guilford Press.

Nathanson, D. L. (1987c). The shame/pride axis. In H. B. Lewis (Ed.), *The role of shame in symptom formation* (pp. 183–205). Hillsdale, NJ: Erlbaum.

Nicholls, J. G. (1978). The development of concepts of effort and ability, perception of academic attainment, and the understanding that difficult tasks require more ability. *Child Development, 49,* 800–814.

Niedenthal, P., Tangney, J. P., & Gavanski, I. (1994). "If only I weren't" versus "If only I hadn't": Distinguishing shame and guilt in counterfactual thinking. *Journal of Personality and Social Psychology, 67,* 585–595.

O'Connor, L. E., Berry, J. W., Inaba, D., & Weiss, J. (1994). Shame, guilt, and depression in men and women in recovery from addiction. *Journal of Substance Abuse Treatment, 11,* 503–510.

O'Connor, L. E., Berry, J. W., & Weiss, J. (1999). Interpersonal guilt, shame and psychological problems. *Journal of Social and Clinical Psychology, 18,* 181–203.

O'Connor, L. E., Berry, J. W., Weiss, J., Bush, M., & Sampson, H. (1997). Interpersonal guilt: The development of a new measure. *Journal of Clinical Psychology, 53,* 73–89.

Osgood, C. E., & Tannenbaum, P. H. (1955). The principle of congruity in the prediction of attitude change. *Psychological Review, 62,* 42–55.

Otterbacher, J. R., & Munz, D. C. (1973). State–trait measure of experiential guilt. *Journal of Consulting and Clinical Psychology, 40,* 115–121.

Patterson, G. R. (1982). *Coercive family process.* Eugene, OR: Castalia Press.

Perlman, M. (1958). An investigation of anxiety as related to guilt and shame. *Archives of Neurology and Psychiatry, 80,* 752–759.

Petersen, D. A., Barlow, D. H., & Tangney, J. P. (1995, August). *Interpersonal perception and metaperception associated with shame-proneness and guilt-proneness.* Poster presented at the annual meeting of the American Psychological Association, New York City.

Phares, E. J., & Erkine, N. (1984). The measurement of selfism. *Educational and Psychological Measurement, 44,* 597–608.

Piaget, J. (1952). *The origins of intelligence in children.* New York: International Universities Press.

Piers, G., & Singer, A. (1953). *Shame and guilt.* Springfield, IL: Thomas.

Potter-Efron, R. T. (1989). *Shame, guilt and alcoholism: Treatment issues in clinical practice.* New York: Haworth Press.

Pulakos, J. (1996). Family environment and shame: Is there a relationship? *Journal of Clinical Psychology, 52,* 617–623.

Raskin, R. N., & Hall, C. S. (1979). A narcissistic personality inventory. *Psychological Reports, 45,* 590.

Raskin, R. N., & Hall, C. S. (1981). The Narcissistic Personality Inventory: Alternate form reliability and further evidence of construct validity. *Journal of Personality Assessment, 45,* 159–162.

Raskin, R. N., & Novacek, J. (1989). An MMPI description of the narcissistic personality. *Journal of Personality Assessment, 53,* 66–88.

Raskin, R. N., & Shaw, R. (1988). Narcissism and the use of personal pronouns. *Journal of Personality Assessment, 56,* 393–404.

Raskin, R. N., & Terry, H. (1988). A principal-components analysis of the Narcissistic Personality Inventory and further evidence of its construct validity. *Journal of Personality and Social Psychology, 54,* 890–902.

Retzinger, S. R. (1987). Resentment and laughter: Video studies of the shame–rage spiral. In H. B. Lewis (Ed.), *The role of shame in symptom formation* (pp. 151–181). Hillsdale, NJ: Erlbaum.

Robins, C. J. (1988). Attributions and depression: Why is the literature so inconsistent? *Journal of Personality and Social Psychology, 54,* 880–889.

Rodin, J., Silberstein, L., & Striegel-Moore, R. (1985). Women and weight: A normative discontent. In T. B. Sondregger (Ed.), *Psychology and gender: Nebraska symposium on motivation, 1984* (pp. 267–307). Lincoln: University of Nebraska Press.

Rogers, C. R. (1961). *On becoming a person.* Boston: Houghton Mifflin.

Rogers, C. R. (1975). The necessary and sufficient conditions of therapeutic personality change. *Journal of Consulting Psychology, 21,* 95–103.

Rosenberg, K. L. (1998). The socialization of shame and guilt. *Dissertation Abstracts International: Section B. The Sciences and Engineering, 58,* 5673.

Rosenberg, K. L., Tangney, J. P., Denham, S., Leonard, A. M., & Widmaier, N. (1994a). *Socialization of Moral Affect—Child Form (SOMA-C).* George Mason University, Fairfax, VA.

Rosenberg, K. L., Tangney, J. P., Denham, S., Leonard, A. M., & Widmaier, N. (1994b). *Socialization of Moral Affect—Parent of Children Form (SOMA-PC).* George Mason University, Fairfax, VA.

Rosenberg, M. (1965). *Society and the adolescent self-image.* Princeton, NJ: Princeton University Press.

Rugel, R. P. (1997). *Husband-focused marital therapy.* Springfield, IL: Thomas.

Saarni, C. (1999). *The development of emotional competence.* New York: Guilford Press.

Sanftner, J. L., Barlow, D. H., Marschall, D. E., & Tangney, J. P. (1995). The relation of shame and guilt to eating disorders symptomotology. *Journal of Social and Clinical Psychology, 14,* 315–324.

Schaefer, D. A. (2000). The difference between shame-prone and guilt-prone persons on measures of anxiety, depression and risk of alcohol abuse. *Dissertation Abstracts International: Section A. Humanities and Social Sciences, 60,* 2389.

Scheff, T. J. (1987). The shame–rage spiral: A case study of an interminable quarrel. In H. B. Lewis (Ed.), *The role of shame in symptom formation* (pp. 109–149). Hillsdale, NJ: Erlbaum.

Scheff, T. J. (1997). *Emotions, the social bond, and human reality.* Cambridge, UK: Cambridge University Press.

Schneidman, E. S. (1968, July). Classification of suicidal phenomena. *Bulletin of Suicidology*, pp. 1–9.

Schore, A. N. (1991). Early superego development: The emergence of shame and narcissistic affect regulation in the practicing period. *Psychoanalysis and Contemporary Thought, 14*, 187–250.

Schulman, M., & Mekler, E. (1985). *Bringing up a moral child*. New York: Addison-Wesley.

Seidman, S. N., & Rieder, R. O. (1994). A review of sexual behavior in the United States. *American Journal of Psychiatry, 151*, 330–341.

Seligman, M. E. P., Abramson, L. Y., Semmel, A., & von Baeyer, C. (1979). Depressive attributional style. *Journal of Abnormal Psychology, 88*, 242–247.

Sherman, L. W. (1993). Defiance, deterrence, and irrelevance: A theory of the criminal sanction. *Journal of Research in Crime and Delinquency, 30*, 445–473.

Shiffler, J. B. (1998). The relationship between guilt- and shame-proneness and Rorschach indices of psychological functioning. *Dissertation Abstracts International: Section B. The Sciences and Engineering, 58*, 6247.

Shilts, R. (1987). *And the band played on: Politics, people, and the AIDS epidemic*. New York: St. Martin's Press.

Simons, R. L., Whitbeck, L. B., Conger, R. D., & Wu, C. I. (1991). Intergenerational transmission of harsh parenting. *Developmental Psychology, 27*, 159–171.

Siomopoulus, V. (1988). Narcissistic personality disorder: Clinical features. *American Journal of Psychotherapy, 42*, 240–253.

Skoe, E. E., & Gooden, A. (1993). Ethic and care and real-life moral dilemma content in male and female early adolescents. *Journal of Early Adolescence, 13*, 154–167.

Skoe, E. E., Pratt, M. W., Matthews, M., & Curror, S. E. (1996). The ethic of care: Stability over time, gender differences, and correlates in mid- to late adulthood. *Psychology and Aging, 11*, 280–292.

Smetana, J. G. (1989). Toddlers' social interactions in the context of moral and conventional transgressions in the home. *Developmental Psychology, 25*, 499–508.

Smetana, J. G., Schlagman, N., & Adams, P. W. (1993). Preschool children's judgments about hypothetical and actual transgressions. *Child Development, 64*, 202–214.

Smith, C. A., & Ellsworth, P. C. (1985). Patterns of cognitive appraisal in emotion. *Journal of Personality and Social Psychology, 48*, 813–838.

Smith, R. L. (1972). The relative proneness to shame or guilt as an indicator of defensive style. *Dissertation Abstracts International, 33*, 2823B.

Snyder, M. (1974). The self monitoring of expressive behavior. *Journal of Personality and Social Psychology, 30*, 526–537.

Snyder, M., & Cantor, N. (1980). Thinking about ourselves and others: Self-monitoring and social knowledge. *Journal of Personality and Social Psychology, 39*, 222–234.

Snyder, M., & Swann, W. B., Jr. (1976). When actions reflect attitudes: The politics of impression management. *Journal of Personality and Social Psychology, 34*, 1034–1042.

Soechting, I., Skoe, E. E., & Marcia, J. E. (1994). Care-oriented moral reasoning and prosocial behavior: A question of gender or sex role orientation. *Sex Roles, 31*, 131–147.

Solomon, R. S. (1982). Validity of the MMPI Narcissistic Personality Disorder Scale. *Psychological Reports, 50*, 463–466.

Spielberger, C. D., Gorsuch, R. L., & Lushene, R. E. (1970). *Manual for the State–Trait Anxiety Inventory*. Palo Alto, CA: Consulting Psychologists Press.

Spielberger, C. D., Johnson, E. H., Russell, S., Crane, R. S., Jacobs, G., & Worder, T. J. (1985). The experience and expression of anger: Construction and validation of an Anger Expression Scale. In M. A. Chesney & R. H. Rosenman (Eds.), *Anger and hostility in cardiovascular and behavioral disorders* (pp. 5–30). New York: Hemisphere.

Stadter, M. (1996). *Object relations brief therapy*. Northvale, NJ: Aronson.

Stegge, H., & Ferguson, T. J. (1990). *Child–Child Attribution and Reaction Survey (C-CARS)*. Utah State University, Logan.

Stiller, N. J., & Forrest, L. (1990). An extension of Gilligan and Lyons' investigation of morality: Gender differences in college students. *Journal of College Student Development, 31*, 54–63.

Straus, M., Gelles, R., & Steinmetz, S. K. (1980). *Behind closed doors: Violence in the American family*. Garden City, NY: Anchor Press.

Sugarman, D. B., & Hotaling, G. T. (1989). Violent men in intimate relationships: An analysis of risk markers. *Journal of Applied Social Psychology, 19*, 1034–1048.

Tangney, J. P. (1989). *Shame and guilt in young adulthood: A qualitative analysis*. Poster presented at the annual meeting of the American Psychological Society, Arlington, VA.

Tangney, J. P. (1990). Assessing individual differences in proneness to shame and guilt: Development of the self-conscious affect and attribution inventory. *Journal of Personality and Social Psychology, 59*, 102–111.

Tangney, J. P. (1991). Moral affect: The good, the bad, and the ugly. *Journal of Personality and Social Psychology, 61*, 598–607.

Tangney, J. P. (1992). Situational determinants of shame and guilt in young adulthood. *Personality and Social Psychology Bulletin, 18*, 199–206.

Tangney, J. P. (1993a). Shame-based anger: Seeds of dysfunctional responses to interpersonal conflict. In R. K. Hason (Chair), *Guilt and shame: Legal, social, and mental health perspectives*. Symposium conducted at the annual meeting of the American Psychological Association, Toronto, Ontario, Canada.

Tangney, J. P. (1993b). Shame and guilt. In C. G. Costello (Ed.), *Symptoms of depression* (pp. 161–180). New York: Wiley.

Tangney, J. P. (1994). The mixed legacy of the super-ego: Adaptive and maladaptive aspects of shame and guilt. In J. M. Masling & R. F. Bornstein (Eds.), *Empirical perspectives on object relations theory* (pp. 1–28). Washington, DC: American Psychological Association.

Tangney, J. P. (1995a). Recent advances in the empirical study of shame and guilt. *American Behavioral Scientist, 38*, 1132–1145.

Tangney, J. P. (1995b). Shame and guilt in interpersonal relationships. In J. P. Tangney & K. W. Fischer (Eds.), *Self-conscious emotions: The psychology of shame, guilt, embarrassment, and pride* (pp. 114–139). New York: Guilford Press.

Tangney, J. P. (1995c). Tales from the dark side of shame: Further implications for interpersonal behavior and adjustment. In R. Baumeister & D. Wegner (Chairs), *From bad to worse: Problematic responses to negative affect*. Symposium conducted at the annual meeting of the Society for Experimental Social Psychology, Washington, DC.

Tangney, J. P. (1996). Conceptual and methodological issues in the assessment of shame and guilt. *Behaviour Research and Therapy, 34*, 741–754.

Tangney, J. P. (2000, July). *Couples in conflict: Constructive vs. destructive responses to everyday anger*. Paper presented at the annual meeting of the International Society for Research on Aggression, Valencia, Spain.

Tangney, J. P., Barlow, D. H., Borenstein, J., & Marschall, D. (2001). *Couples in conflict: Implications of shame for the (mis)management of anger in intimate relationships*. Manuscript in preparation.

Tangney, J. P., Barlow, D. H., Wagner, P. E., Marschall, D., Borenstein, J. K., Sanftner, J., Mohr, T., & Gramzow, R. (1996). Assessing individual differences in constructive vs. destructive responses to anger across the lifespan. *Journal of Personality and Social Psychology, 70,* 780–796.

Tangney, J. P., Burggraf, S. A., Hamme, H., & Domingos, B. (1988). *The Self-Conscious Affect and Attribution Inventory (SCAAI).* Bryn Mawr College, Bryn Mawr, PA.

Tangney, J. P., Burggraf, S. A., & Wagner, P. E. (1995). Shame-proneness, guilt-proneness, and psychological symptoms. In J. P. Tangney & K. W. Fischer (Eds.), *Self-conscious emotions: The psychology of shame, guilt, embarrassment, and pride* (pp. 343–367). New York: Guilford Press.

Tangney, J. P., & Dearing, R. L. (in press). Gender differences in morality. In J. M. Masling & R. F. Bornstein (Eds.), *Empirical perspectives on psychoanalytic theory* (Vol. 10). Washington, DC: American Psychological Association.

Tangney, J. P., Dearing, R. L., Wagner, P. E., & Gramzow, R. (2000). *The Test of Self-Conscious Affect-3 (TOSCA-3).* George Mason University, Fairfax, VA.

Tangney, J. P., Fee, R., Reinsmith, C., Bowling, L., & Yerington, T. (1997). *Beliefs about the self: Implications for psychological adjustment and moral affective style.* Poster presented at the annual meeting of the Society for Experimental Social Psychology, Toronto, Ontario, Canada.

Tangney, J. P., Ferguson, T. J., Wagner, P. E., Crowley, S. L., & Gramzow, R. (1996). *The Test of Self-Conscious Affect-2 (TOSCA-2).* George Mason University, Fairfax, VA.

Tangney, J. P., Marschall, D. E., Rosenberg, K., Barlow, D. H., & Wagner, P. E. (1994). *Children's and adults' autobiographical accounts of shame, guilt and pride experiences: An analysis of situational determinants and interpersonal concerns.* Unpublished manuscript.

Tangney, J. P., Miller, R. S., & Flicker, L. (1992). *A quantitative analysis of shame and embarrassment.* Poster presented at the annual meeting of the American Psychological Association, Washington, DC.

Tangney, J. P., Miller, R. S., Flicker, L., & Barlow, D. H. (1996). Are shame, guilt and embarrassment distinct emotions? *Journal of Personality and Social Psychology, 70,* 1256–1269.

Tangney, J. P., Niedenthal, P. M., Covert, M. V., & Barlow, D. H. (1998). Are shame and guilt related to distinct self-discrepancies?: A test of Higgins' (1987) hypothesis. *Journal of Personality and Social Psychology, 75,* 256–268.

Tangney, J. P., Wagner, P. E., & Barlow, D. H. (2001). *The relation of shame and guilt to empathy: An intergenerational study.* Manuscript in preparation.

Tangney, J. P., Wagner, P. E., Barlow, D. H., Marschall, D. E., & Gramzow, R. (1996). The relation of shame and guilt to constructive vs. destructive responses to anger across the lifespan. *Journal of Personality and Social Psychology, 70,* 797–809.

Tangney, J. P., Wagner, P. E., Burggraf, S. A., Gramzow, R., & Fletcher, C. (1990). *The Test of Self-Conscious Affect for Children (TOSCA-C).* George Mason University, Fairfax, VA.

Tangney, J. P., Wagner, P. E., Burggraf, S. A., Gramzow, R., & Fletcher, C. (1991). *Children's shame-proneness, but not guilt-proneness, is related to emotional and behavioral maladjustment.* Poster presented at the annual meeting of the American Psychological Society, Washington, DC.

Tangney, J. P., Wagner, P. E., Fletcher, C., & Gramzow, R. (1992). Shamed into anger?: The relation of shame and guilt to anger and self-reported aggression. *Journal of Personality and Social Psychology, 62,* 669–675.

Tangney, J. P., Wagner, P. E., Gavlas, J., & Gramzow, R. (1991a). *The Test of Self-Conscious Affect for Adolescents (TOSCA-A).* George Mason University, Fairfax, VA.

Tangney, J. P., Wagner, P. E., Gavlas, J., & Gramzow, R. (1991b). *The Anger Response Inventory for Adolescents (ARI-Adol).* George Mason University, Fairfax, VA.

Tangney, J. P., Wagner, P. E., & Gramzow, R. (1989). *The Test of Self-Conscious Affect (TOSCA).* George Mason University, Fairfax, VA.

Tangney, J. P., Wagner, P. E., & Gramzow, R. (1992). Proneness of shame, proneness to guilt, and psychopathology. *Journal of Abnormal Psychology, 103*, 469–478.

Tangney, J. P., Wagner, P. E., Hansbarger, A., & Gramzow, R. (1991). *The Anger Response Inventory for Children (ARI-C)*. George Mason University, Fairfax, VA.

Tangney, J. P., Wagner, P. E., Marschall, D., & Gramzow, R. (1991). *The Anger Response Inventory (ARI)*. George Mason University, Fairfax, VA.

Tannen, D. (1990). *You just don't understand: Women and men in conversation*. New York: Morrow.

Tavris, C. (1992). *The mismeasure of woman*. New York: Simon & Schuster.

Taylor, G. (1985). *Pride, shame and guilt: Emotions of self-assessment*. Oxford, UK: Clarendon Press.

Taylor, S. E., Klein, L. C., Lewis, B. P., Gruenewald, T. L., Gurung, R. A., & Updegraff, J. A. (2000). Biobehavioral responses to stress in females: Tend-and-befriend, not fight-or-flight. *Psychological Review, 107*, 411–429.

Tesser, A. (1999). Toward a self-evaluation maintenance model of social behavior. In R. F. Baumeister (Ed.), *The self in social psychology* (pp. 446–460.) Philadelphia: Psychology Press.

Tesser, A., & Campbell, J. (1980). Self-definition: The impact of relative performance and similarity of others. *Social Psychology Quarterly, 43*, 341–347.

Tesser, A., & Campbell, J. (1983). Self-definition and self-evaluation maintenance. In J. Suls & A. Greewald (Eds.), *Social psychological perspectives on the self* (Vol. 2, pp. 1–31). Hillsdale, NJ: Erlbaum.

Tomkins, S. (1963). *Affect, imagery, consciousness: Vol. 2. The negative affects*. New York: Springer.

Tooke, W. S., & Ickes, W. (1988). A measure of adherence to conventional morality. *Journal of Social and Clinical Psychology, 6*, 310–334.

Turner, J. E. (1998). *An investigation of shame reactions, motivation, and achievement in a difficult college course*. Unpublished doctoral dissertation, University of Texas, Austin.

Vagg, J. (1998). Delinquency and shame. *British Journal of Criminology, 38*, 247–264.

Wahl, O. F. (1995). *Media madness: Public images of mental illness*. New Brunswick, NJ: Rutgers University Press.

Walker, L. (1984). Sex differences in the development of moral reasoning: A critical review. *Child Development, 55*, 677–691.

Walker, L. (1986). Sex differences in the development of moral reasoning: A rejoinder to Baumrind. *Child Development, 57*, 522–527.

Wallbott, H. G., & Scherer, K. R. (1995). Cultural determinants in experiencing shame and guilt. In J. P. Tangney & K. W. Fischer (Eds.), *Self-conscious emotions: The psychology of shame, guilt, embarrassment, and pride* (pp. 465–487). New York: Guilford Press.

Wark, G. R., & Krebs, D. L. (1996). Gender and dilemma differences in real-like moral judgment. *Developmental Psychology, 32*, 220–230.

Watson, P. J., Grisham, S. D., Trotter, M. V., & Biderman, M. D. (1984). Narcissism and empathy: Validity evidence for the Narcissistic Personality Inventory. *Journal of Personality Assessment, 48*, 301–305.

Watson, P. J., Taylor, D., & Morris, R. J. (1987). Narcissism, sex roles, and self-functioning. *Sex Roles, 16*, 335–350.

Weiner, B. (1986). Attribution, emotion, and action. In R. M. Sorrentino & E. T. Higgins (Eds.), *Handbook of motivation and cognition: Foundations of social behavior* (pp. 281–312). New York: Guilford Press.

Weiner, I. B. (1998). *Principles of psychotherapy*. New York: Wiley.

Weiss, R. L., & Halford, W. K. (1996). Managing marital therapy. In V. B. Van Hasselt &

M. Hersen (Eds.), *Sourcebook of psychological treatment manuals for adult disorders* (pp. 489–537). New York: Plenum Press.

Wells, M., Glickauf-Hughes, C., & Jones, R. (1999). Codependency: A grass roots construct's relationship to shame-proneness, low self-esteem, and childhood parentification. *American Journal of Family Therapy, 27*, 63–71.

Wells, M., & Jones, R. (2000). Childhood parentification and shame-proneness: A preliminary study. *American Journal of Family Therapy, 28*, 19–27.

Whitbeck, L. B., Hoyt, D. R., Simons, R. L., Conger, R. D., Elder, G. H., Lorenz, F. O., & Huck, S. (1992). Intergenerational continuity of parental rejection and depressed affect. *Journal of Personality and Social Psychology, 63*, 1036–1045.

White, J. (1994). Individual characteristics and social knowledge in ethical reasoning. *Psychological Reports, 75*, 627–649.

White, J., & Manolis, C. (1997). Individual differences in ethical reasoning among law students. *Social Behavior and Personality, 25*, 19–48.

Wicker, F. W., Payne, G. C., & Morgan, R. D. (1983). Participant descriptions of guilt and shame. *Motivation and Emotion, 7*, 25–39.

Widom, C. S. (1987). Child abuse, neglect, and adult behavior: Research design and findings on criminality, violence, and child abuse. *American Journal of Orthopsychiatry, 59*, 355–367.

Widom, C. S. (1989). Does violence beget violence? A critical examination of the literature. *Psychological Bulletin,106*, 3–28.

Wilchins, R. (1997). *Read my lips: Sexual subversion and the end of gender.* New York: Firebrand Books.

Williams, C., & Bybee, J. (1994). What do children feel guilty about? Developmental and gender differences. *Developmental Psychology, 30*, 617–623.

Witkin, H. A., Lewis, H. B., Hertzman, M., Machover, K., Meissner, P. B., & Wapner, S. (1954). *Personality through perception: An experimental and clinical study.* New York: Harper.

Witkin, H. A., Lewis, H. B., & Weil, E. (1968). Affective reactions and patient–therapist interactions among more differentiated and less differentiated patients early in therapy. *Journal of Nervous and Mental Disease, 146*, 193–208.

Wurmser, L. (1987). Shame: The veiled companion of narcissism. In D. L. Nathanson (Ed.), *The many faces of shame* (pp. 64–92). New York: Guilford Press.

Yarrow, M. R., Waxler, C. Z., & Scott, P. M. (1971). Child effects on adult behavior. *Developmental Psychology, 5*, 300–311.

Zahn-Waxler, C., Kochanska, G., Krupnick, J., & Mayfield, A. (1988). *Coding manual for children's interpretations of interpersonal distress and conflict.* Bethesda, MD: Laboratory of Developmental Psychology, National Institute of Mental Health.

Zahn-Waxler, C., Kochanska, G., Krupnick, J., & McKnew, D. (1990). Patterns of guilt in children of depressed and well mothers. *Developmental Psychology, 26*, 51–59.

Zahn-Waxler, C., & Robinson, J. (1995). Empathy and guilt: Early origins of feelings of responsibility. In J. P. Tangney & K. W. Fischer (Eds.), *Self-conscious emotions: The psychology of shame, guilt, embarrassment, and pride* (pp. 143–173). New York: Guilford Press.

Zamble, E., & Quinsey, V. L. (1997). *The criminal recidivism process.* New York: Cambridge University Press.

AUTHOR INDEX

SUBJECT INDEX

(*"n"* indicates a note)

Academic failure, children, 187–189
Adaptive function
  guilt, 118, 119, 122–125
  shame, 125–127
Adjective checklists
  advantages and limitations, 37, 38, 50
  description of, 34, 37, 38
  internal consistency, 41, 51n2
  psychopathology studies, 119
  scenario-based measures distinction, 39, 40
Adolescents
  anger response, 100, 103, 104, 111n1
  assessment instruments, 35, 36, 40, 100
  moral emotions and moral behavior, 134–137
  moral standards development, 142
  shame- versus guilt-proneness stability, 145, 146
Aggression, 90–111 (*see also* Anger)
  anger distinction, 98, 99
  assessment, 97–103
  children's expression of, 97
  in couple conflicts, 160–162
  longitudinal study, 135
  sex differences, 109
  shame-proneness link, 97–107, 135
AIDS-related shame, 168, 169
Alcohol use/abuse, 134–137
Alpha coefficient, 41, 51n2, 238
Altruism
  empathy link, 81

moral reasoning relationship, 131–133
and prosocial reasoning, 133
Anger, 90–111
  aggression distinction, 98, 99
  assessment, 97–103
  behavioral responses, 100–102
  in children, 186, 187
  constructive responses, 97–107
  in couple conflicts, 160–162
  destructive responses, 97–107, 160–162
  developmental shift, 111n1
  empathy shaping, 107
  empirical studies, 93–110
  and externalization of blame, 91–95
  gender differences, 109
  guilt-proneness expression of, 95–107
  and intentions, 100, 101
  nonaggressive responses, 101–103
  potential benefits, 99
  shame dynamics, 91–94
    interpersonal relationship implications, 94–95
    in parenting, 185–187
  shame-proneness studies, 96–107
  and shame–rage spiral, 162
  and situation-specific shame feelings, 97–110
Anger Held in Scale, 102
Anger Response Inventories, 99–103
Anthropological perspective, 13–18
Anxiety, 120, 202
Anxiety Attitude Survey, 34

265